Mercho Raushdi Shoemaker & Dilley
Inc.

1315 N. Arlington
Suite 100
 Indpls., In

Diagnostic Ultrasound
Principles, Instrumentation, and Exercises

Second Edition

Frederick W. Kremkau, Ph.D.

Professor and Director
Center for Medical Ultrasound
Bowman Gray School of Medicine
Winston-Salem, North Carolina

Grune & Stratton, Inc.
Harcourt Brace Jovanovich, Publishers
Orlando   New York   San Diego   Boston   London
San Francisco   Tokyo   Sydney   Toronto

Grune & Stratton, Inc.
Orlando, FL 32887

Distributed in the United Kingdom by
Grune & Stratton, Ltd.
24/28 Oval Road, London NW 1

Library of Congress Catalog Number 84-47817
International Standard Book Number 0-8089-1643-2
Printed in the United States of America

86 87 88   10 9 8 7 6 5 4 3 2

To Lil and Jonathan

Contents

Acknowledgments   x
Preface   xi

Chapter 1.   **Introduction**   **1**

    1.1   Motivation
    1.2   The Big Picture

Chapter 2.   **Ultrasound**   **5**

    2.1   Introduction
    2.2   Waves and Sound
    2.3   Pulsed Ultrasound
    2.4   Amplitude and Intensity
    2.5   Attenuation
    2.6   Review

Chapter 3.   **Reflection and Scattering**   **32**

    3.1   Introduction
    3.2   Perpendicular Incidence
    3.3   Oblique Incidence
    3.4   Scattering
    3.5   Range Equation
    3.6   Review

Chapter 4.   **Transducers and Sound Beams**   48

    4.1   Introduction
    4.2   Transducers
    4.3   Beams and Focusing
    4.4   Resolution and Useful Frequency Range
    4.5   Review

Chapter 5.   **Static Imaging Instruments**   74

    5.1   Introduction
    5.2   Pulser
    5.3   Receiver
    5.4   Memory
    5.5   Display
    5.6   Review

Chapter 6.   **Dynamic Imaging Instruments**   112

    6.1   Introduction
    6.2   Real-Time Transducers
    6.3   Real-Time Displays
    6.4   Review

Chapter 7.   **Doppler Instruments**   123

    7.1   Introduction
    7.2   Doppler Effect
    7.3   Continuous-Wave Instruments
    7.4   Pulsed Instruments
    7.5   Spectral Analysis
    7.6   Review

Chapter 8.   **Artifacts**   139

    8.1   Introduction
    8.2   Artifacts
    8.3   Review

Chapter 9.   **Performance Measurements**   154

    9.1   Introduction
    9.2   Imaging Performance
    9.3   Beam Profile and Frequency Spectrum
    9.4   Acoustic Output
    9.5   Review

Chapter 10.   **Bioeffects and Safety**   166

    10.1   Introduction
    10.2   Bioeffects
    10.3   Safety
    10.4   Review

Chapter 11. **Misconceptions and Errors** 178

11.1 Literature Errors
11.2 Setting Things Straight

Chapter 12. **Summary** 192

Glossary 209

Answers to Exercises in the Text 218

Appendix A. **Symbols List** 237

Appendix B. **Equations List** 239

Appendix C. **Mathematics** 243

C.1 Algebra
C.2 Trigonometry
C.3 Logarithms and Scientific Notation
C.4 Decibels
C.5 Binary Numbers
C.6 Units

Appendix D. **Physics Concepts** 266

D.1 Mechanics
D.2 Energy

Answers to Exercises in the Appendixes 272

References 275

Index 279

Acknowledgments

The author gratefully acknowledges helpful discussions and criticism from P. L. Carson, F. Dunn, L. A. Frizzel, B. B. Goldberg, A. Goldstein, J. C. Hobbins, G. R. Leopold, J. J. Nanasi, W. L. Nyborg, W. D. O'Brien, Jr., K. J. W. Taylor, P. N. T. Wells, J. A. Zagzebski, and M. C. Ziskin; the instruction and wise counsel of his teachers, E. L. Carstensen, H. G. Flynn, and R. Gramiak; and the assistance of Andrea D'Aurio in manuscript preparation.

Preface

This book is for sonographers and sonologists who need basic knowledge of the physical principles and instrumentation of diagnostic ultrasound. Its purpose is to explain how diagnostic ultrasound works. It does not describe how to perform diagnostic examinations or to interpret the results, except to point out artifact possibilities. Little background in mathematics and physics is assumed. Help in these areas is available in Appendixes C and D, which may be studied before beginning Chapter 1. Several hundred exercises are provided to check progress, strengthen concepts, and provide practice for registry and specialty board examinations. Answers are given starting on page 218. Exercises at the end of each chapter may be used as pretests to determine knowledge in specific subject areas. Terms defined in the glossary are boldface when first mentioned in the text. Many statements in this book are simplifications of the actual situation. They are used for simplicity and brevity. Some clarification of this is given in Chapter 11.

This second edition contains major new and expanded material in the areas of digital instrumentation, real-time transducers, Doppler imaging and analysis, artifacts, and misconceptions. Equations are given in both verbal and symbolic form. An equals sign with an asterisk indicates that the equation is specifically for soft tissues. An equals sign with two asterisks indicates that the equation is specifically for perpendicular incidence at a boundary. Superscript numbers refer to citations in the reference list, starting on page 275.

Diagnostic Ultrasound

Chapter 1

Introduction

There are five reasons for learning the material in this book:

1. to learn how diagnostic **ultrasound** works[1]*
2. to become knowledgeable about possible artifacts
3. to prepare for registry and specialty board examinations
4. to prepare for instrumentation performance measurement procedures
5. to become aware of safety and risk considerations

1.1 Motivation

Ultrasound is useful in medical diagnosis primarily because it provides a method for visualizing internal body tissues and structures. The visualization method consists of two steps:

1. sending short **pulses** of ultrasound into the body
2. using **reflections** received from various tissues to produce an image of internal structures

   The heart of the method is the interaction between ultrasound and tissues (Figure 1.1). The effects of the tissues on the ultrasound (**acoustic propagation properties**) are discussed in Chapters 2 and 3. This is the aspect of the interaction that is useful in diagnosis. The adjective

1.2 The Big Picture

*Boldface words are defined in the glossary starting on page 209. A superscript number refers to a citation in the References section starting on page 275.

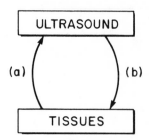

Figure 1.1. The interaction between ultrasound and tissues. (a) The effects of tissues on ultrasound are called the acoustic propagation properties of tissues. They are what make ultrasound useful as a diagnostic tool. (b) The effects of ultrasound on tissues are called the bioeffects. They must be considered when discussing the safety of the diagnostic method.

acoustic refers to **sound. Propagation** means progression or travel. The effects of the ultrasound on tissues (bioeffects) are considered in Chapter 10. The diagnostic ultrasound visualization method is described in Figure 1.2. Chapter 4 discusses how ultrasound is generated and received. The instruments that control the generation of ultrasound and display the received reflections are described in Chapters 5 and 6. Measurements for determining the proper function of instruments are discussed in Chapter 9.

In addition to anatomic imaging, ultrasound provides a method for detecting motion and flow. The instruments that do this are described in Chapter 7.

References 2–8 are other sources for the study of diagnostic ultrasound physical principles.

Exercises

1.2.1. The diagnostic ultrasound visualization method has two parts:
1. Sending short _____ of _____ into the body.
2. Using _____ received from various tissues to produce an _____ of internal structures.

1.2.2. The heart of the diagnostic method is the interaction between _____ and _____ .

1.2.3. The effects of the tissues on ultrasound are called _____ propagation properties of tissues. They make ultrasound useful as a _____ tool.

1.2.4. The effects of ultrasound on tissues are called _____ .

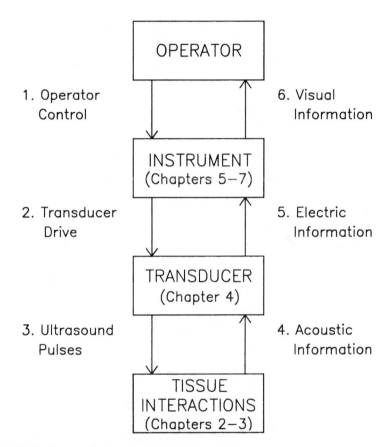

Figure 1.2. The diagnostic ultrasound visualization method. 1. The operator controls the operation of the instrument. 2. The instrument produces electrical voltages that drive the transducer. 3. The transducer produces ultrasound pulses that travel into the body and interact with the tissues. 4. The reflections generated in the tissues bring acoustic information to the transducer. 5. The transducer sends to the instrument electric information corresponding to the received reflections. 6. The instrument converts the electric information to a visual form that is useful for medical diagnosis.

1.2.5. Match the following to decribe the steps of the diagnostic ultrasound visualization method:

a. the operator controls the _____ .

b. The instrument drives the _____ .

c. The transducer produces ultrasound _____ .

d. The transducer receives _____ information.

e. The instrument receíves _____ information.

f. The operator receives _____information.

1. acoustic
2. visual
3. transducer
4. instrument
5. electric
6. pulses

1.2.6. Match the means by which the components of the diagnostic ultrasound visualization method interact:

a. operator and instrument: _____

b. instrument and transducer: _____

c. transducer and tissue: _____

1. electric voltages
2. ultrasound pulses
3. hand/eye

Chapter 2

Ultrasound

Ultrasound can provide information concerning internal body structures and motion. It is like the ordinary sound that we hear except that it has a **frequency** (discussed in the next section) higher than that to which the human hearing system responds.

2.1 Introduction

Sound is a **wave.** A wave is a propagating (progressive or traveling) variation in quantities called **wave variables.** Waves carry **energy,*** not matter, from one place to another. Sound (Figure 2.1) is one particular type of wave. It is a propagating variation in quantities called **acoustic variables.** These acoustic variables include **pressure, density, temperature,** and **particle motion.** A **particle** is a small portion of the **medium** through which the sound is traveling. Unlike light waves and radio waves, sound requires a medium through which to travel. It cannot pass through a vacuum. Sound is a mechanical **longitudinal wave** in which back-and-forth particle motion is parallel to the direction of wave travel.

Like all waves, sound is described by a few parameters. These are frequency, **period, wavelength, propagation speed, amplitude,** and **intensity.** Frequency, period, amplitude, and intensity are determined

2.2 Waves and Sound

*This and other basic physics terms are discussed in Appendix D.

5

Figure 2.1. Sound is traveling variations of acoustic variables (pressure, density, temperature, particle motion).

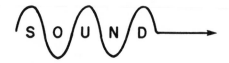

by the sound source. Propagation **speed** is determined by the medium, and wavelength is determined by both the source and the medium.

Recall that sound is a traveling variation. Frequency describes how many complete variations **(cycles)** an acoustic variables goes through in a second. Take pressure as an example of an acoustic variable. Pressure may start at its normal (undisturbed) value, increase to a maximum value, return to normal, decrease to a minimum value, and return to normal. This describes a complete cycle of variation of pressures as an acoustic variable. As a sound wave travels past some point, this cycle is repeated over and over. The number of times that it occurs in 1 second is called the frequency (Figure 2.2).

Frequency units* include the **hertz (Hz)** and **megahertz (MHz).** One hertz is one cycle per second or one complete variation per second. One megahertz is 1,000,000 Hz. Table C.6 gives unit prefixes. Sound with a frequency of 20,000 Hz or higher is called ultrasound because it is beyond the frequency range of human hearing. This is analogous to ultraviolet light, which is higher in frequency than human eyes can see. Frequency will be important later when image resolution and **half-intensity depth** are considered.

Period is the time that it takes for one cycle to occur (Figure 2.3). It is the reciprocal of frequency. Period units include seconds (s) and microseconds (μs). One microsecond is one-millionth of a second (0.000001 s). Period will be important when pulsed ultrasound is considered in Section 2.3. A list of common periods is given in Table 2.1. Period decreases as frequency increases.[†]

$$\text{period (μs)} = \frac{1}{\text{frequency (MHz)}} \qquad T = \frac{1}{f}$$

Wavelength is the length of space over which one cycle occurs (Figure 2.4). Its units include meters (m) and millimeters (mm). One millimeter is one-thousandth of a meter (0.001 m). Wavelength will be important when image resolution is considered.

*Units are discussed in Appendix C.

†For convenient reference, symbols are compiled in Appendix A and equations in Appendix B. Equations and algebra are discussed in Appendix C. In parentheses are abbreviations representing units (Appendix C) appropriate for each quantity.

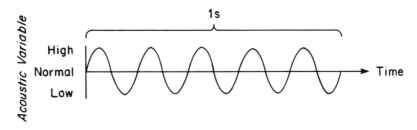

Figure 2.2. Frequency is the number of complete variations (cycles) that an acoustic variable goes through in 1 s. In this figure, five cycles occur each second; the frequency is five complete variations per second, or 5 Hz.

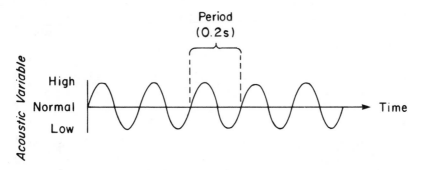

Figure 2.3. Period is the time it takes for one cycle to occur. In this figure, each cycle occurs in 0.2 s. The period is 0.2 s, and the frequency is the reciprocal of 0.2 s, or 5 Hz.

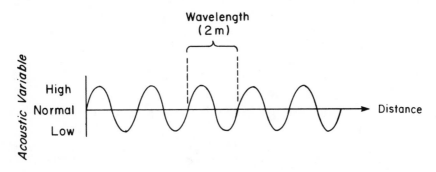

Figure 2.4. Wavelength is the length of space over which one cycle occurs. In this figure, each cycle covers 2 m. The wavelength is 2 m. This figure differs from Figures 2.2 and 2.3 in that the horizontal axis represents distance rather than time.

Table 2.1
Common Ultrasound Periods and Wavelengths* in Tissue

Frequency (MHz)	Period (μs)	Wavelength (mm)
1.00	1.00	1.54
2.25	0.44	0.68
3.50	0.29	0.44
5.00	0.20	0.31
7.50	0.13	0.21
10.0	0.10	0.15

*Assume propagation speed 1.54 mm/μs.

Propagation speed is the speed with which a wave moves through a medium. It is the speed with which a *particular value* of an acoustic variable moves. An easily identified value of an acoustic variable is its maximum value. The speed with which this maximum value moves through a medium is the propagation speed (Figure 2.5). It depends on the medium but *not* on the frequency. Wavelength is equal to propagation speed divided by frequency.

$$\text{wavelength (mm)} = \frac{\text{propagation speed (mm/μs)}}{\text{frequency (MHz)}} \qquad \lambda = \frac{c}{f}$$

An example of the relationship among frequency, wavelength, and propagation speed may be seen by comparing Figures 2.2, 2.4, and 2.5 (see the legend for Figure 2.5). Propagation speed units include meters per second (m/s) and millimeters per microsecond (mm/μs). One millimeter per microsecond equals 1000 m/s. Wavelength decreases as frequency increases.

Propagation speed is determined by the density and **stiffness** (hardness) of the medium. Density is the concentration of matter (**mass** per unit volume). Stiffness is the resistance of a material to compression. Propagation speed increases if the stiffness is increased or if the density is *decreased* (a surprising fact for many students).* As an illustration, the propagation speed in brass is lower than that in aluminum even though the density of brass is approximately three times that of aluminum.

In general, propagation speeds through gases are low, propagation speeds through liquids are higher, and propagation speeds through solids are the highest. This *increasing* sequence is not caused by the increasing density (which produces a decreasing propagation speed) but by the increasing stiffness. This is because the stiffness differences are larger than the density differences. The average propagation speed

*Common misconceptions are discussed in Chapter 11.

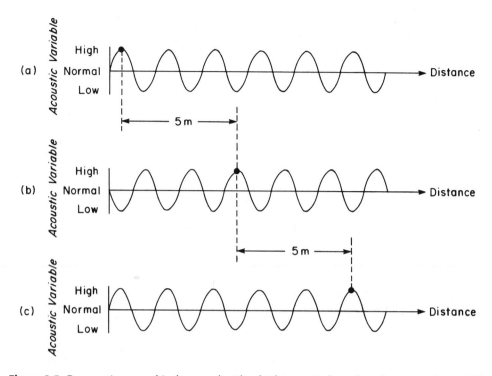

Figure 2.5. Propagation speed is the speed with which a particular value of an acoustic variable moves. The movement of a maximum (identified by the dot) is shown in this figure. Example (b) is 0.5 s after (a). Example (c) is 0.5 s after (b) and 1 s after (a). The maximum (dot) moves 5 m in 0.5 s and 10 m in 1 s. The propagation speed is 10 m/s. The propagation speed in this figure (10 m/s) divided by the frequency in Figure 2.2 (5 Hz) equals the wavelength in Figure 2.4 (2 m).

in soft tissues is 1540 m/s or 1.54 mm/μs. Values for specific tissues are given in Table 2.2. In lung (which contains gas), the propagation speed is lower than in other soft tissues, generally in the range of 0.3–1.2 mm/μs.* The propagation speed in bone (a solid) is higher than that in soft tissue, generally in the range of 2–4 mm/μs.* Goss et al.[10] give propagation speed values for various tissues. Values for fat (about 1.44 mm/μs) are significantly lower than the soft-tissue average. Propagation speed is important because imaging instruments make use of it in generating the display. This is discussed in Chapter 5. Using the average propagation speed for soft tissue, wavelength is as follows.†

*In Section 2.5 we will see that ultrasound does not penetrate lung or bone well, so that these differing propagation speeds are normally not of concern.

†An equals sign with an asterisk indicates that the equation is specifically for soft tissues.

Table 2.2
Propagation Speeds in Soft Tissues.[9]

Tissue	Propagation Speed (mm/μs)
Fat	1.44
Brain	1.51
Liver	1.56
Kidney	1.56
Muscle	1.57
Soft-tissue average	1.54

For soft tissues	
wavelength (mm) $\overset{*}{=} \dfrac{1.54}{\text{frequency (MHz)}}$	$\lambda \overset{*}{=} \dfrac{1.54}{f}$

A list of common wavelengths is given in Table 2.1.

Impedance is defined as density multiplied by propagation speed. It will be important for the discussion of reflections in Chapter 3.

impedance (rayl) = density (kg/m^3) $\times$ propagation speed (m/s)	$z = \rho c$

Its unit is the **rayl.** Impedance is determined by the density and stiffness of a medium. It increases if the density is increased or if the stiffness is increased. Recall that propagation speed also depends on density and stiffness, but in a different way. Impedance does *not* depend on frequency.

Typical values for frequency, period, wavelength, propagation speed, and impedance are given in Table 2.7 in Section 2.6.

Exercises

2.2.1. A wave is a traveling variation in quantities called
_____ _____ .

2.2.2. Sound is a traveling variation in quantities called
_____ _____ .

2.2.3. Ultrasound is sound with a frequency of
_____ Hz or higher.

2.2.4. Acoustic variables include _____ ,
_____ , _____ , and
_____ _____ .

2.2.5. Which of the following frequencies are in the ultrasound range? (More than one correct answer.)
   a. 15 Hz
   b. 15,000 Hz
   c. 15 MHz
   d. 30,000 Hz
   e. 0.04 MHz

2.2.6. Which of the following are acoustic variables? (More than one correct answer.)
   a. pressure
   b. frequency
   c. propagation speed
   d. period
   e. particle motion

2.2.7. Frequency is a measure of how many _____ an acoustic variable goes through in a second.

2.2.8. The unit of frequency is the _____ , which is abbreviated _____ .

2.2.9. Period is the _____ that it takes for one cycle to occur.

2.2.10. Period is the _____ of frequency.

2.2.11. Wavelength is the length of _____ over which one cycle occurs.

2.2.12. Propagation speed is the speed with which a _____ moves through a medium.

2.2.13. Wavelength is equal to _____ _____ divided by _____ .

2.2.14. Propagation speed is determined by the _____ and _____ of a medium.

2.2.15. Propagation speed increases if
   a. density is increased
   b. density is decreased
   c. stiffness is increased
   d. a and c
   e. b and c

2.2.16. The average propagation speed in soft tissues is _____ m/s or _____ mm/μs.

2.2.17. Propagation speed is determined by
a. frequency
b. amplitude
c. wavelength
d. period
e. medium

2.2.18. Place the following in order of increasing sound propagation speed:
a. gas
b. solid
c. liquid

2.2.19. The wavelength of 1-MHz ultrasound in soft tissues is _____ mm.

2.2.20. Wavelength in soft tissues _____ as frequency increases.

2.2.21. It takes _____ µs for ultrasound to travel 1.54 cm in soft tissue.

2.2.22. Propagation speed in bone is _____ than in soft tissues.

2.2.23. Sound travels fastest in
a. air
b. helium
c. water
d. iron
e. a vacuum

2.2.24. Solids have higher propagation speeds than liquids because they have higher
a. density
b. stiffness

2.2.25. The propagation speeds through mercury and fat are approximately the same, even though the density of mercury is approximately 15 times that of fat. This means that the stiffness of mercury must be much _____ than that of fat.

2.2.26. Sound is a _____ _____ wave.

2.2.27. If propagation speed is doubled (a different medium) and frequency is held constant, the wavelength is _____ .

2.2.28. If wavelength in a given medium at a given frequency is 2 mm and the frequency is doubled, the wavelength becomes _____ mm.

2.2.29. If frequency in soft tissue is doubled, propagation speed is
_____ .

2.2.30. Waves carry _____ from one place to
another.

2.2.31. From given values for propagation speed and frequency,
which of the following can be calculated?
a. amplitude
b. period
c. wavelength
d. a and b
e. b and c

2.2.32. If two media have the same stiffness but different densities,
the one with the higher density will have the higher
propagation speed. True or false?

2.2.33. If two media have the same density but different stiffnesses,
the one with the higher stiffness will have the higher
propagation speed. True or false?

2.2.34. If the density is 1000 kg/m^3 and the propagation speed is
1.54 mm/µs, the impedance is _____ rayls.

2.2.35. If two media have the same stiffness but different densities,
the one with the higher density will have the higher
impedance. True or false?

2.2.36. If two media have the same density but different stiffnesses,
the one with the higher stiffness will have the higher
impedance. True or false?

2.2.37. Impedance is _____ multiplied by
_____ _____ .

The terms discussed earlier (frequency, period, wavelength, and propagation speed) describe a **continuous wave (cw).** For diagnostic ultrasound imaging, continuous-wave sound is not commonly used. Instead, short pulses of sound are used. This is called **pulsed ultrasound.** It is produced by applying **electric pulses** to the **transducer** (see Chapter 4). Ultrasound pulses are described by some additional parameters that have not yet been introduced.

Pulse repetition frequency is the number of pulses occurring in a second (Figure 2.6). Its units include the hertz (Hz) and **kilohertz (kHz).** One kilohertz is 1000 Hz.

The **pulse repetition period** is the time from the beginning of one pulse to the beginning of the next (Figure 2.7). Its units include seconds (s) and milliseconds (ms). One millisecond is one-thousandth of a sec-

2.3
Pulsed
Ultrasound

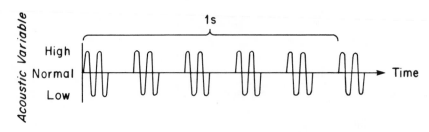

Figure 2.6. Pulse repetition frequency is the number of pulses occurring in 1 s. In this figure, five pulses (containing two cycles each) occur in 1 s; thus the pulse repetition frequency is 5 Hz.

ond (0.001 s). The pulse repetition period is the reciprocal of pulse repetition frequency.

$$\text{pulse repetition period (ms)} = \frac{1}{\text{pulse repetition frequency (kHz)}} \quad \bigg| \quad PRP = \frac{1}{PRF}$$

Pulse duration is the time that it takes for a pulse to occur (Figure 2.7). It is equal to the period times the number of cycles in the pulse. Its units include seconds (s) and microseconds (μs).

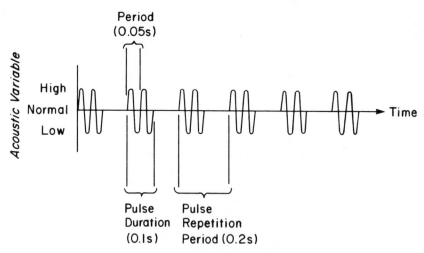

Figure 2.7. The pulse repetition period is the time from the beginning of one pulse to the beginning of the next. In this figure, the pulse repetition period is 0.2 s. Therefore, the pulse repetition frequency is 5 Hz. Pulse duration is the time that it takes for one pulse to occur. It is equal to the period times the number of cycles in the pulse. In this figure, pulse duration is 0.1 s. Since two cycles occur in a 0.1-s pulse in this figure, the period is 0.05 s, and the frequency is 20 Hz. The duty factor is the fraction of time that the sound is actually on. It is pulse duration divided by pulse repetition period. The duty factor in this figure is 0.5.

14

pulse duration (μs) = number of cycles in the pulse × period (μs)	$PD = n \times T$
$= \dfrac{\text{number of cycles in the pulse}}{\text{frequency (MHz)}}$	$PD = \dfrac{n}{f}$

The second equation is derived from the first by substituting 1/frequency for period. Pulse duration decreases if the number of cycles is decreased or if frequency is increased.

Duty factor is the fraction of time that sound (in the form of pulses) is actually on. It is calculated by dividing the pulse duration by the pulse repetition period. The duty factor is unitless. It will be important when intensities are discussed in Section 2.4.

$\text{duty factor} = \dfrac{\text{pulse duration (μs)}}{\text{pulse repetition period (ms)} \times 1000}$	$DF = \dfrac{PD}{PRP \times 1000}$
$\text{duty factor} = \dfrac{\text{pulse duration (μs)} \times \text{pulse repetition frequency (kHz)}}{1000}$	$DF = \dfrac{PD \times PRF}{1000}$

The second equation is derived from the first by substituting 1/pulse repetition frequency for pulse repetition period. By multiplying the duty factor by 100, the result is expressed in percent.

Spatial pulse length is the length of space over which a pulse occurs (Figure 2.8). It is equal to the wavelength times the number of cycles in the pulse. Its units include meters (m) and millimeters (mm). It will be an important quantity when **axial resolution** is discussed in Section 4.4.

spatial pulse length (mm) = number of cycles in the pulse × wavelength (mm)	$SPL = n \times \lambda$
spatial pulse length (mm) = $\dfrac{\text{number of cycles in the pulse} \times \text{propagation speed (mm/μs)}}{\text{frequency (MHz)}}$	$SPL = \dfrac{n \times c}{f}$
For soft tissues: spatial pulse length (mm) $\overset{*}{=} \dfrac{\text{number of cycles in the pulse} \times 1.54}{\text{frequency (MHz)}}$	$SPL \overset{*}{=} \dfrac{n \times 1.54}{f}$

The second equation is derived from the first by substituting propagation speed/frequency for wavelength.

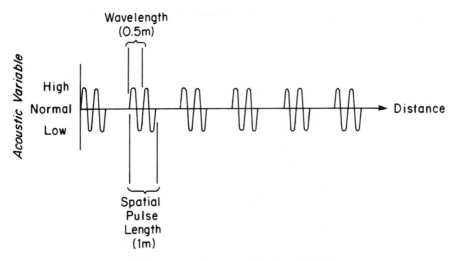

Figure 2.8. Spatial pulse length is the length of space over which a pulse occurs. It is equal to wavelength times the number of cycles in the pulse. In this figure, wavelength is 0.5 m, there are two cycles in each pulse, and spatial pulse length is 0.5 times 2, or 1 m. This figure differs from Figures 2.6 and 2.7 in that the horizontal axis represents distance rather than time.

The propagation speed for pulses is the same as that for continuous waves in a given medium. Frequency within pulses (as opposed to pulse repetition frequency) is the same as that for continuous waves. For pulses, frequency gives the number of cycles per second assuming continuous waves (even though this assumption is not correct for pulsed ultrasound). Therefore, 1-MHz pulsed ultrasound with a duty factor of 0.1 percent will have only 1000 cycles per second (because the quiet time between pulses eliminates 99.9 percent of the cycles) even though the frequency implies that there are 1 million cycles per second.

Typical values for pulse repetition frequency, pulse repetition period, pulse duration, duty factor, and spatial pulse length are given in Table 2.7 in Section 2.6.

Exercises

2.3.1. The abbreviation cw stands for _____
_____ .

2.3.2. Pulsed ultrasound is ultrasound in the form of repeated short _____ .

2.3.3. Pulse repetition frequency is the number of _____occurring in 1 s.

2.3.4. Pulsed ultrasound is produced by applying electric _____to the transducer.

2.3.5. The pulse repetition _____is the time from the beginning of one pulse to the beginning of the next.

2.3.6. The pulse repetition period is the _____of pulse repetition frequency.

2.3.7. Pulse duration is the _____for a pulse to occur.

2.3.8. Spatial pulse length is the _____of _____over which a pulse occurs.

2.3.9. _____ _____ is the fraction of time that pulsed ultrasound is actually on.

2.3.10. Pulse duration equals the number of the cycles in the pulse times _____ .

2.3.11. Spatial pulse length equals the number of cycles in the pulse times _____ .

2.3.12. The duty factor of continuous-wave sound is _____ .

2.3.13. If the wavelength is 2 mm, the spatial pulse length for a three-cycle pulse is _____mm.

2.3.14. The spatial pulse length in soft tissue for a four-cycle pulse of frequency 3 MHz is _____mm.

2.3.15. The pulse duration in soft tissue for a four-cycle pulse of frequency 3 MHz is _____μs.

2.3.16. For a 1-kHz pulse repetition frequency, the pulse repetition period is _____ms.

2.3.17. For problems 2.3.15 and 2.3.16 together, the duty factor is _____ .

2.3.18. How many cycles are there in 1 second of continuous-wave 5 MHz ultrasound?
a. 5
b. 500
c. 5,000
d. 5,000,000
e. none of the above

2.3.19. How many cycles are there in 1 second of pulsed 5 MHz ultrasound with duty factor .001?
a. 5
b. 500
c. 5,000
d. 5,000,000
e. none of the above

2.3.20. In problem 2.3.19, how many cycles were eliminated by pulsing?

a. 100 percent
b. 99.9 percent
c. 99 percent
d. 50 percent
e. 1 percent

2.4 Amplitude and Intensity

The rate at which cycles occur in time (frequency), the time required for each cycle (period), the space over which a cycle occurs (wavelength), and the speed at which the cycles move (propagation speed) have been described. The magnitude of the variations will now be considered. This will give some idea of the **strength** of the sound. Amplitude and intensity are the parameters that are relevant here.

Amplitude is the maximum variation that occurs in an acoustic variable. It is the maximum value minus the normal (undisturbed) value (Figure 2.9). Amplitude is given in units appropriate for the acoustic variable considered.

Intensity is the **power** in a wave divided by the area over which the power is spread.

$$\text{intensity (W/cm}^2) = \frac{\text{power (W)}}{\text{area (cm}^2)} \qquad I = \frac{P}{A}$$

Power is discussed in Appendix D. Power units include watts (W) and milliwatts (mW). If the total power across a sound beam is divided by the **beam area,** the spatial average intensity is calculated. This is discussed later in this section. **Sound beams** and beam area will be discussed in Section 4.3. Beam area units are centimeters squared (cm^2). Intensity units include watts per centimeter squared (W/cm^2) and others listed in Table C.7. Intensity is an important parameter in describing the sound that is produced and received by diagnostic instrumentation (see Chapter 5) and in discussing bioeffects and safety (see Chapter 10). It may be illustrated by analogy with sunlight incident on dry leaves. Sunlight will not normally ignite the leaves, but if the same power is concentrated into a small area (increased intensity) by **focusing** with a magnifying glass, the leaves can be ignited. An effect is therefore produced by increasing the intensity even though the power remains the same.

It will be seen in Section 4.3 that beam area is determined in part by the size and **operating frequency** of the sound source chosen. For a given beam power, intensity will be determined by the beam area resulting from the choice of sound source.

Intensity is proportional to the amplitude squared. Thus, if amplitude is doubled, intensity is quadrupled. If amplitude is halved, intensity is quartered.

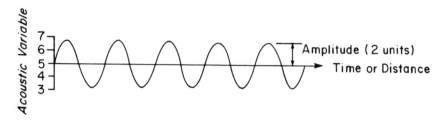

Figure 2.9. Amplitude is the maximum amount of variation that occurs in an acoustic variable. It is equal to the maximum value of the variable minus the normal (undisturbed) value. In this figure, the amplitude is seven (maximum value) minus five (normal value); the amplitude is two units.

Because intensity is not uniform across a sound beam (Figure 2.10) and, in the case of pulsed ultrasound, is not uniform in time (Figure 2.11), four intensities must be considered. For spatial considerations either the spatial peak (SP) or spatial average (SA) value may be used. These are related by the **beam uniformity ratio.** The beam uniformity ratio is defined as the spatial peak intensity divided by the spatial average intensity.

$$\text{spatial average intensity (W/cm}^2) = \frac{\text{spatial peak intensity (W/cm}^2)}{\text{beam uniformity ratio}} \qquad I_{SA} = \frac{I_{SP}}{BUR}$$

For temporal (time) considerations, either the temporal peak (TP) value or temporal average (TA) value may be used. These are related by the duty factor.

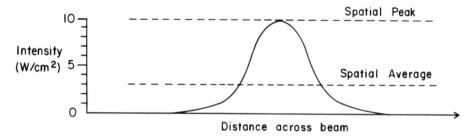

Figure 2.10. Intensity is a function of distance across the beam. In this figure the spatial peak intensity (at the beam center) is 10 W/cm^2, the spatial average is 3 W/cm^2, and the beam uniformity ratio is 3.3. In addition to varying across the beam, intensity varies along the direction of the beam.

19

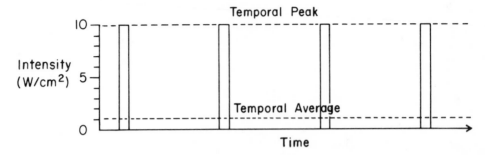

Figure 2.11. Intensity as a function of time for pulsed ultrasound. Temporal peak intensity (10 W/cm²) is the intensity when the sound is actually on. Temporal average intensity (1 W/cm²) is the intensity that results when this is averaged over time. In this figure, the duty factor is 0.1.

temporal average intensity (W/cm²) = duty factor × temporal peak intensity (W/cm²)	$I_{TA} = DF \times I_{TP}$

If the sound is continuous instead of pulsed, the duty factor is unity, and the temporal peak and temporal average intensities are equal to each other. The four intensities resulting from spatial and temporal considerations are spatial-average–temporal-average (SATA) intensity, spatial-peak–temporal-average (SPTA) intensity, spatial-average–temporal peak (SATP) intensity, and spatial-peak–temporal-peak (SPTP) intensity. These are related to one another as shown in Table 2.3.

The pulses shown in Figures 2.6 and 2.11 have constant amplitude and intensity during each pulse. Pulses used in diagnostic ultrasound are typically like that shown in Figure 2.12. In this case the peak intensity occurring within each pulse is called the temporal peak intensity. The intensity averaged over the pulse duration is called the pulse average intensity (it is called temporal peak intensity elsewhere in this section, where pulses are assumed to have constant intensity within them, as in Figure 2.11).

Example 2.4.1 The SATA intensity is 1 mW/cm², the beam uniformity ratio is 10, and the duty factor is 0.002. Calculate SPTA, SATP, and SPTP intensities.

$$\text{SPTA intensity} = \text{SATA intensity} \times \text{beam uniformity ratio}$$

$$= 1 \times 10 = 10 \text{ mW/cm}^2$$

$$\text{SATP intensity} = \frac{\text{SATA intensity}}{\text{duty factor}}$$

$$= \frac{1}{0.002} = 500 \text{ mW/cm}^2$$

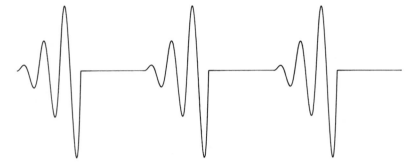

Figure 2.12. Ultrasound pulses used in imaging. These pulses have cycles of differing amplitudes. They are produced by electrical shock excitation of a damped transducer (see Chapter 4 and Figure 4.5 for details).

$$\text{SPTP intensity} \; = \; \frac{\text{SATA intensity} \times \text{ beam uniformity ratio}}{\text{duty factor}}$$

$$= \; \frac{1 \times 10}{0.002} \; = \; 5000 \text{ mW/cm}^2 \; = \; 5 \text{ W/cm}^2$$

SATA intensity is the lowest of the four, and SPTP intensity is the highest. SPTA and SATP intensities have intermediate values with SATP normally being the greater of the two.

Table 2.3
Process of Conversion from One Intensity to Another*

To Convert	to	Multiply (Divide) by	and by
SATA	SPTA	beam uniformity ratio	1
	SATP	1	(duty factor)
	SPTP	beam uniformity ratio	(duty factor)
SPTA	SATA	(beam uniformity ratio)	1
	SATP	(beam uniformity ratio)	(duty factor)
	SPTP	1	(duty factor)
SATP	SATA	1	duty factor
	SPTA	beam uniformity ratio	duty factor
	SPTP	beam uniformity ratio	1
SPTP	SATA	(beam uniformity ratio)	duty factor
	SPTA	1	duty factor
	SATP	(beam uniformity ratio)	1

*For example, to convert SATA to SPTP, multiply by beam uniformity ratio and divide by duty factor. SATA: spatial-average–temporal-average intensity. SPTA: spatial-peak–temporal-average intensity. SATP: spatial-average–temporal-peak intensity. SPTP: spatial-peak–temporal-peak intensity.

Exercises

2.4.1. Amplitude is the maximum _____ that occurs in an acoustic variable.

2.4.2. Intensity is the _____ in a wave divided by _____ .

2.4.3. The unit for intensity is _____ .

2.4.4. Intensity is proportional to the square of _____ .

2.4.5. If power is doubled and area remains unchanged, intensity is _____ .

2.4.6. If area is doubled and power remains unchanged, intensity is _____ .

2.4.7. If both power and area are doubled, intensity is _____ .

2.4.8. If amplitude is doubled, intensity is _____ .

2.4.9. If a sound beam has a power of 10 mW and a beam area of 2 cm^2, the spatial average intensity is _____ mW/cm^2

2.4.10. The beam uniformity ratio is the spatial _____ intensity divided by the spatial _____ intensity.

2.4.11. The duty factor is equal to temporal _____ intensity divided by temporal _____ intensity.

2.4.12. Which of the following intensities are equal for continuous-wave sound?
a. spatial peak and average
b. temporal peak and average
c. spatial peak and temporal average
d. spatial average and temporal average
e. none of the above

2.4.13. If the SATA intensity is 1 mW/cm^2, the beam uniformity ratio is 3, and the duty factor is 0.001, calculate the following intensities:
a. SPTA: _____ mW/cm^2
b. SATP: _____ W/cm^2
c. SPTP: _____ W/cm^2

2.4.14. If pulsed ultrasound is on 50 percent of the time (duty factor = 0.5) and temporal peak intensity is 4 mW/cm^2, temporal average intensity is _____ mW/cm^2.

2.4.15. If the maximum value of an acoustic variable is 10 units and the normal (undisturbed) value is 7 units, the amplitude is _____ units. The minimum value of the acoustic variable is _____ .

The terms discussed previously (frequency, period, wavelength, propagation speed, amplitude, and intensity) describe sound waves. Another term, **attenuation,** is needed before sound reflection is considered (Chapter 3). It is important to understand attenuation because it must be compensated for by the diagnostic instrument (Section 5.3).

2.5 Attenuation

For an unfocused beam (beams and focus are discussed in Chapter 4) in any real medium such as tissue, amplitude and intensity will decrease as the sound travels through the medium. This reduction in amplitude and intensity as sound travels is called attenuation (Figure 2.13). It encompasses **absorption** (conversion of sound to heat), reflection (Sections 3.2 and 3.3), and **scattering** (Section 3.4). Attenuation units are **decibels (dB).** The **attenuation coefficient** is the attenuation per unit length of sound travel. Its units are decibels per centimeter (dB/cm). See Appendix C for a discussion of decibels. The longer the path over which the sound travels, the greater the attenuation.

$$\text{attenuation (dB)} = \frac{\text{attenuation coefficient (dB/cm)}}{\times \text{ path length (cm)}} \qquad a = a_c l$$

The attenuation coefficient increases with increasing frequency. Persons who live in apartments or dormitories experience this fact when they hear mostly the bass notes through the wall from a neighbor's sound system. For soft tissues, attenuation coefficients are given in Table 2.4. A simple approximation is that soft tissue, on the average, has 1 dB of attenuation per centimeter for each megahertz of frequency (Table 2.5). Therefore, the average attenuation coefficient in decibels per centimeter for soft tissues is approximately equal to the frequency in megahertz. In order to calculate the attenuation in decibels simply multiply the frequency in megahertz (which is approximately equal to the attenuation coefficient in dB/cm) by the path length in centimeters, and the result is the attenuation in decibels.

$$\text{For soft tissues:} \\ \text{attenuation (dB)} \overset{*}{=} \text{frequency (MHz)} \times \text{path length (cm)} \qquad a \overset{*}{=} f \times l$$

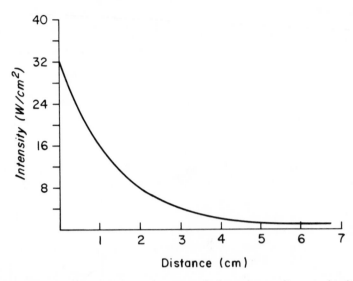

Figure 2.13. Attenuation of sound as it travels through a medium. In this figure, the intensity decreases by 50 percent for each 1 cm of travel. This corresponds to an attenuation coefficient of 3 dB/cm.

Table 2.4
Attenuation Coefficients in Tissues.[9,10]

	Attenuation Coefficient (dB/cm)	
Tissue	at 1 MHz	at 10 MHz
Fat	0.6	7.6
Brain	0.6	8.4
Liver	0.7	9.4
Kidney	0.9	10.7
Muscle	1.0	12.6
Heart	1.1	13.3
Soft tissue average*	0.8	10.1

*Fat, liver, kidney, muscle.

Table 2.5
Average Attenuation Coefficients in Tissue

Frequency (MHz)	Average Attenuation Coefficient for Soft Tissue (dB/cm)	Intensity Reduction in 1-cm Path (%)	Intensity Reduction in 10-cm Path (%)
1	1	21	90.0
2	2	37	99.0
3	3	50	99.9
5	5	68	99.999
7	7	80	99.99999
10	10	90	99.99999999

The intensity ratio corresponding to that number of decibels may be obtained from Table C.2. This ratio is equal to the fraction of the intensity (at the beginning of the path) that remains at the end of the path. If the intensity at the beginning is known, the intensity at the end may be found by multiplying by the intensity ratio. A summary of this three-step process is:

1. Frequency (MHz) times path length (cm) yields attenuation (dB).
2. Find the intensity ratio in Table C.2 for the decibel value calculated in Step 1.
3. The intensity ratio times the intensity at the start of the path equals the intensity at the end of the path.

Example 2.5.1. If 2-MHz ultrasound at 10 mW/cm² SATA intensity is applied to a soft-tissue surface, what is the SATA intensity 1.5 cm into the tissue? The frequency (MHz) multiplied by the path length (cm) is equal to 3. The attenuation is 3 dB. From Table C.2 it can be found that 3 dB corresponds to an intensity ratio of 0.5. Thus, 50 percent of the intensity remains after the sound travels through this path. The intensity ratio (0.5) times the SATA intensity at the beginning of the path (10 mW/cm²) gives the SATA intensity at the end of the path (5 mW/cm²).

Attenuation is higher in lung than in other soft tissues. In bone it is higher than in soft tissues. Lung and bone attenuations are not linearly dependent on frequency.

A practical consequence of attenuation is that it limits the depth at which images can be obtained. A useful parameter related to this is the half-intensity depth. It is defined as the depth at which intensity is reduced to 50 percent (3 dB) of its original value. It therefore is also the distance over which 50 percent of the original intensity is lost. The half-intensity depth decreases as frequency increases. It is useful when considering to what depths in tissue imaging may be accomplished. However, half-intensity depth does not imply that imaging cannot be performed beyond this depth. It normally can. The two are related, so that if half-intensity depth decreases (for example, because of an increase in frequency) imaging depth also decreases. Table 2.6 lists half-intensity depths for various frequencies in soft tissue.

$$\text{half-intensity depth (cm)} = \frac{3}{\text{attenuation coefficient (dB/cm)}} \qquad D = \frac{3}{a_c}$$

For soft tissues:

$$\text{half-intensity depth} \overset{*}{=} \frac{3}{\text{frequency (MHz)}} \qquad D \overset{*}{=} \frac{3}{f}$$

Table 2.6
Average Half-Intensity Depths in Tissue

Frequency (MHz)	Half-Intensity Depth (cm)
1.00	3.0
2.25	1.3
3.50	0.9
5.00	0.6
7.50	0.4
10.0	0.3

Exercises

2.5.1. Attenuation is the reduction in _____ and _____ as a wave travels through a medium.

2.5.2. Attenuation consists of _____ , _____ , and _____ .

2.5.3. The attenuation coefficient is attenuation per unit _____ of sound travel.

2.5.4. The attenuation and attenuation coefficient are given in the units _____ and _____ , respectively.

2.5.5. For soft tissues, there is approximately _____ dB of attenuation per centimeter for each megahertz of frequency.

2.5.6. For soft tissues, the attenuation coefficient at 3 MHz is approximately _____ .

2.5.7. The attenuation coefficient in soft tissue _____ as frequency increases.

2.5.8. For soft tissue, if frequency is doubled, attenuation is _____ ; if path length is doubled, attenuation is _____ ; if both frequency and path length are doubled, attenuation is _____ .

2.5.9. If frequency is doubled and path length is halved, attenuation is _____ .

2.5.10. Absorption is the conversion of _____ to _____ .

2.5.11. Can the absorption be greater than the attenuation in a given medium at a given frequency? _____ .

2.5.12. Is attenuation in bone higher or lower than in soft tissue? _____ .

2.5.13. For average soft tissue, the attenuation is such that for each 1.5 cm traveled, a 2-MHz sound intensity is reduced by _____ percent; the half-intensity depth is _____ cm. For 1 cm and 3 MHz, the reduction is _____ percent, and the half-intensity depth is _____ cm.

2.5.14. The half-intensity depth for soft tissue at 5 MHz is _____ cm.

2.5.15. The attenuation coefficient for soft tissue at 5 MHz is _____ dB/cm.

2.5.16. The half-intensity depth is three times the reciprocal of the _____ .

2.5.17. The half-intensity depth _____ as frequency increases.

2.5.18. If the intensity of 2-MHz ultrasound entering soft tissue is 2 W/cm^2, the intensity at a depth of 4 cm is _____ W/cm^2. The half-intensity depth is _____ cm.

2.5.19. If the intensity of 20-MHz ultrasound entering soft tissue is 2 W/cm^2, the intensity at a depth of 4 cm is _____ W/cm^2.

2.5.20. The half-intensity depth in soft tissues at 3.5 MHz is _____ cm.
  a. 0.6
  b. 0.7
  c. 0.8
  d. 0.9
  e. 1.0

Ultrasound is a wave of traveling acoustic variables: pressure, density, temperature, and particle motion. It is described by frequency, period, wavelength, propagation speed, amplitude, intensity, and attenuation. Pulsed ultrasound is described by additional terms: pulse repetition frequency, pulse repetition period, pulse duration, duty factor, and spatial pulse length. Propagation speed and impedance are characteristics of the medium that are determined by density and stiffness. Attenuation increases with frequency and path length. Half-intensity depth decreases with increasing frequency. Four intensities (SATA, SPTA, SATP, and SPTP) are used to describe pulsed ultrasound. The soft-tissue propagation speed is 1.54 mm/μs, and the attenuation coefficient is 1 dB/cm for each megahertz of frequency. Table 2.7 gives typical values for several parameters of diagnostic ultrasound.

2.6 Review

Table 2.7

Diagnostic Ultrasound Parameters in Tissue

Parameter	Typical Value
Frequency	3.5 MHz
Period	0.3 µs
Wavelength	0.4 mm
Propagation speed	1.54 mm/µs
Impedance	1,630,000 rayl
Pulse repetition frequency	1 kHz
Pulse repetition period	1 ms
Cycles per pulse	3
Pulse duration	1 µs
Spatial pulse length	1 mm
Duty factor	0.001
Spatial peak temporal average intensity	1 mW/cm^2
Spatial peak temporal peak intensity	1 W/cm^2
Attenuation coefficient	3 dB/cm
Half-intensity depth	1 cm

Exercises

2.6.1. Which of the following is a characteristic of a medium through which sound is propagating?
  a. impedance
  b. intensity
  c. amplitude
  d. frequency
  e. period

2.6.2. Which of the following applies to continuous-wave sound?
  a. pulse duration
  b. pulse repetition frequency
  c. frequency
  d. beam uniformity ratio
  e. c and d

2.6.3. Match the following:
  a. frequency: _____
  b. period: _____
  c. wavelength: _____
  d. propagation speed: _____
  e. amplitude: _____

  1. time per cycle
  2. maximum variation per cycle
  3. length per cycle
  4. cycles per second
  5. speed of a wave through a medium

2.6.4. Match the following:

    a. wavelength: _____
    b. duty factor: _____
    c. intensity: _____
    d. beam uniformity ratio:

    _____

1. $\dfrac{\text{SPTA intensity}}{\text{SATA intensity}}$
2. $\dfrac{\text{propagation speed}}{\text{frequency}}$
3. $\dfrac{\text{pulse duration}}{\text{pulse repetition period}}$
4. $\dfrac{\text{power}}{\text{beam area}}$

2.6.5. Match the following:

    a. period: _____
    b. pulse repetition period:

    _____

    c. impedance: _____
    d. propagation speed:

    _____

    e. half-intensity depth:

    _____

    f. pulse duration: _____
    g. spatial pulse length:

    _____

1. density × propagation speed
2. frequency × wavelength
3. $\dfrac{1}{\text{frequency}}$
4. $\dfrac{1}{\text{pulse repetition frequency}}$
5. $\dfrac{3}{\text{attenuation coefficient}}$
6. number of cycles in the pulse × wavelength
7. number of cycles in the pulse × period

2.6.6. Match the following quantities with their units (answers may be used more than once):

    a. frequency: _____
    b. wavelength: _____
    c. period: _____
    d. propagation speed: _____
    e. pulse duration: _____
    f. pulse repetition frequency:

    _____

    g. pulse repetition period:

    _____

    h. intensity: _____
    i. attenuation: _____
    j. attenuation coefficient: _____
    k. power: _____
    l. beam area: _____
    m. half-intensity depth: _____

1. s
2. mm/μs
3. Hz
4. mm
5. W/cm^2
6. W
7. dB/cm
8. dB
9. cm^2

2.6.7. Match the following (each answer should be used twice):
   a. attenuation coefficient =   1. soft tissues
      1 dB/cm at 1 MHz: _____   2. lung
   b. high attenuation: _____ ,   3. bone

   _____
   c. high propagation speed:

   _____
   d. propagation speed 1.54
      mm/μs _____
   e. low propagation speed: _____

2.6.8. Given the following:
    frequency = 2 MHz
    pulse repetition frequency = 1 kHz
    4 cycles per pulse
    SATA intensity = 1 mW/cm^2
    beam uniformity ratio = 4
    density = 1058 kg/m^3
   Applying these values to a soft-tissue surface, find the
   following:
   a. propagation speed: _____ mm/μs
   b. wavelength: _____ mm
   c. spatial pulse length: _____ mm
   d. period: _____ μs
   e. pulse duration: _____μs
   f. pulse repetition period: _____ ms
   g. duty factor: _____
   h. SPTP intensity at the surface: _____ W/cm^2
   i. attenuation coefficient: _____ dB/cm
   j. half-intensity depth: _____ cm
   k. attenuation from surface to 3 cm depth: _____ dB
   l. intensity ratio corresponding to dB in k:

   _____
   m. SATA intensity at 3 cm depth: _____ mW/cm^2
   n. SPTA intensity at 3 cm depth: _____ mW/cm^2
   o. SATP intensity at 3 cm depth: _____
     mW/cm^2
   p. SPTP intensity at 3 cm depth: _____
     mW/cm^2
   q. impedance: _____ rayls

2.6.9. Which of the following cannot be determined from the
   others?
   a. frequency
   b. period

    c. amplitude
    d. wavelength
    e. propagation speed

2.6.10. Which of the following cannot be determined from the others?
    a. frequency
    b. amplitude
    c. intensity
    d. power
    e. beam area

2.6.11. If density and stiffness are increased, impedance is _____ .

Chapter 3

Reflection and Scattering

3.1 Introduction

In Chapter 2 the propagation of ultrasound through homogeneous media was considered. The usefulness of ultrasound as an imaging tool is primarily the result of reflection and scattering at organ boundaries and scattering within heterogeneous tissues. These phenomena will be considered in this chapter.

3.2 Perpendicular Incidence

Perpendicular incidence (sometimes called normal incidence) occurs when the direction of travel of the ultrasound is **perpendicular** to the boundary between two media (Figure 3.1). If the incidence is not perpendicular, it is called **oblique incidence.** This will be discussed in the next section.

When there is perpendicular incidence, the incident sound may be reflected or transmitted or both (Figure 3.2). Reflected sound travels through medium one in a direction opposite to the incident sound (i.e., the reflected sound returns to the sound source). Transmitted sound moves through medium two in the same direction as the incident sound. The intensities of the reflected sound and transmitted sound depend on the incident intensity and the impedances of the media.

The reflected intensity divided by the incident intensity is called the **intensity reflection coefficient.** The transmitted intensity divided by the incident intensity is called the **intensity transmission coefficient.***

---

*An equation with two asterisks above the equal sign is specifically for perpendicular incidence.

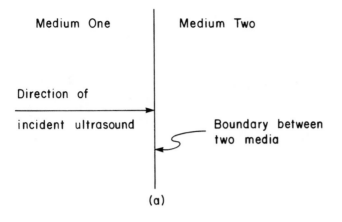

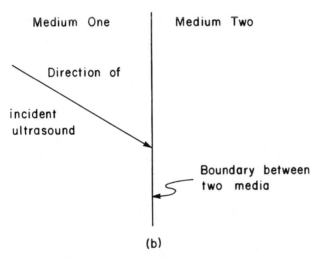

Figure 3.1. Perpendicular incidence (a) and oblique incidence (b) at a boundary between two media.

With perpendicular incidence:	
intensity reflection coefficient $= \dfrac{\text{reflected intensity (W/cm}^2)}{\text{incident intensity (W/cm}^2)}$	$IRC = \dfrac{I_r}{I_i}$
$\overset{..}{=} \left[\dfrac{\text{medium two impedance } - \text{ medium one impedance}}{\text{medium two impedance } + \text{ medium one impedance}} \right]^2$	$\overset{..}{=} \left[\dfrac{Z_2 - Z_1}{Z_2 + Z_1} \right]^2$
intensity transmission coefficient $=$ $\dfrac{\text{transmitted intensity (W/cm}^2)}{\text{incident intensity (W/cm}^2)}$	$ITC = \dfrac{I_t}{I_i}$
$\overset{..}{=} 1 - \text{intensity reflection coefficient}$	$\overset{..}{=} 1 - IRC$

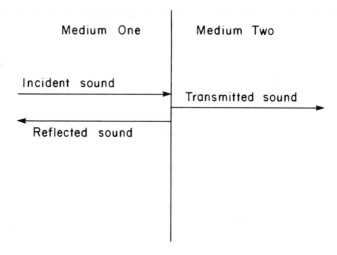

Figure 3.2. Reflection and transmission at a boundary with perpendicular incidence. The lateral offset of transmitted and reflected sound with respect to incident sound is for figure clarity. An actual lateral shift does not occur.

It can be seen that, for perpendicular incidence, if the media impedances are the same, there is no reflected sound, and transmitted intensity is equal to incident intensity. If there is no reflection, the media impedances are equal. It can also be seen that the reflected and transmitted intensities depend not only on the (subtraction) difference between the media impedances but also on their sum (compare Problems 3.2.4 and 3.2.5, where the impedance differences are the same, but the answers are different, and compare Problems 3.2.4 and 3.2.6, where impedance differences are different, but the answers are the same).

Recall that impedance is density times propagation speed. For perpendicular incidence, a reflection is generated at a boundary if the impedances are different. A reflection may be generated when the densities are the same if the propagation speeds are different (see Problem 3.2.10). On the other hand, no reflection may be generated even when the densities are different (see Problem 3.2.11). If there is a large difference between the impedances, there will be almost total reflection (intensity reflection coefficient close to unity). An example of this is an air/soft-tissue boundary (see Problem 3.2.17). For this reason, a **coupling medium** (an oil or a gel) is used to provide a good sound path from the source to the skin during the diagnostic use of ultrasound.

For impedances of 40 and 60 rayls, calculate the intensity reflection *Example* and transmission coefficient. *3.2.1.*

$$\text{intensity reflection coefficient} = \left[\frac{60 - 40}{60 + 40}\right]^2$$

$$= \left[\frac{20}{100}\right]^2 = 0.2^2 = 0.04$$

$$\text{intensity transmission coefficient} = 1 - 0.04 = 0.96$$

The intensity reflection coefficient can be expressed as 4 percent and the intensity transmission coefficient as 96 percent.

If the incident intensity is known, the reflected and transmitted intensities can be calculated by multiplying the incident intensity by the intensity reflection coefficient and the intensity transmission coefficient, respectively.

For Example 3.2.1 if the incident intensity is 10 mW/cm^2 calculate the *Example* reflected and transmitted intensities. *3.2.2.*

From Example 3.2.1, the intensity reflection and transmission coefficients are 0.04 and 0.96, respectively.

$$\text{reflected intensity} = 10 \times 0.04 = 0.4 \text{ mW/cm}^2$$
$$\text{transmitted intensity} = 10 \times 0.96 = 9.6 \text{ mW/cm}^2$$

These coefficients give the fraction of the incident intensity that is reflected or transmitted. By multiplying the coefficients by 100, these fractions are expressed in percent. They must always add up to 1 (or 100 percent).

Exercises

3.2.1. When ultrasound encounters a boundary with perpendicular incidence, the _____ of the tissues must be different to produce a reflection.

3.2.2. With perpendicular incidence, two media _____ and the incident _____ must be known in order to calculate reflected intensity.

3.2.3. With perpendicular incidence, two media _____ must be known in order to calculate the intensity reflection coefficient.

3.2.4. For an incident intensity of 2 mW/cm^2 and impedances of 49 and 51 rayls, the reflected intensity is _____ mW/cm^2, and the transmitted intensity is _____ mW/cm^2.

3.2.5. For an incident intensity of 2 mW/cm^2 and impedances of 99 and 101 rayls, the reflected and transmitted intensities are _____ and _____ mW/cm^2.

3.2.6. For an incident intensity of 2 mW/cm^2 and impedances of 98 and 102 rayls, the reflected and the transmitted intensities are _____ and _____ mW/cm^2.

3.2.7. For an incident intensity of 5 mW/cm^2 and impedances of 45 and 55 rayls, the intensity reflection coefficient is _____ or _____ percent.

3.2.8. For impedances of 45 and 55 rayls, the intensity transmission coefficient is _____ or _____ percent.

3.2.9. For impedances of 45 and 55 rayls, the intensity reflection coefficient is _____ dB.

3.2.10. Given the following:
incident intensity = 1 mW/cm^2
medium one:
   density = 1.0 kg/m^3
   propagation speed = 1350 m/s
medium two:
   density = 1.0 kg/m^3
   propagation speed = 1650 m/s
The reflected intensity is _____ mW/cm^2.

3.2.11. Given the following:
incident intensity = 5 mW/cm^2
medium one:
   density = 1.00 kg/m^3
   propagation speed = 1515 m/s
medium two:
   density = 1.01 kg/m^3
   propagation speed = 1500 m/s
The reflected intensity is _____ mW/cm^2.

3.2.12. Given the following:
incident intensity = 5 mW/cm^2
medium one impedance = 2 rayls
medium two impedance = 0 rayls
The reflected and transmitted intensities are _____ and _____ mW/cm^2.

3.2.13. If the impedances of the media are equal, there is no reflection. True or false?

3.2.14. If the densities of the media are equal, there is no reflection. True or false?

3.2.15. If propagation speeds of the media are equal, there is no reflection. True or false?

3.2.16. The intensity reflection and transmission coefficients depend on whether the sound is traveling from medium one into medium two or vice versa. True or false?

3.2.17. The intensity reflection coefficient at a boundary between soft tissue (impedance 1,630,000 rayls) and air (impedance 400 rayls) is _____ .

3.2.18. A coupling medium is used to eliminate _____ between the sound source and the skin, thus eliminating a strong _____ at the air/skin boundary.

3.2.19. The intensity reflection coefficient at a boundary between fat (impedance 1,380,000 rayls) and muscle (impedance 1,700,000 rayls) is _____ .

3.2.20. The intensity reflection coefficient at a boundary between soft tissue (impedance of 1,630,000 rayls) and bone (impedance 7,800,000 rayls) is _____ .

3.2.21. With perpendicular incidence, the reflected intensity depends on
a. density difference
b. acoustic impedance difference
c. acoustic impedance sum
d. both b and c
e. both a and b

3.3 Oblique Incidence

Oblique incidence occurs when the direction of travel of the incident ultrasound is not perpendicular to the boundary between two media (Figure 3.1). The direction of travel with respect to the boundary is given by the **incidence angle** (for perpendicular incidence, the incidence angle is zero, Section 3.2). The reflected and transmitted directions are given by the **reflection angle** and **transmission angle,** respectively (Figure 3.3). They are related as follows:

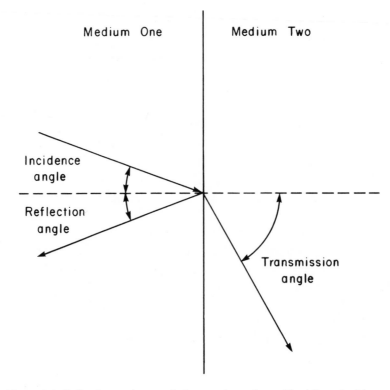

Figure 3.3. Reflection and transmission at a boundary with oblique incidence. Incidence and reflection angles are equal. The transmission angle depends on the incidence angle and the media propagation speeds.

reflection angle (°) = incidence angle (°)	$\Theta_r = \Theta_i$
transmission angle (°) = incidence angle (°) × $\left[\dfrac{\text{medium two propagation speed (mm/}\mu\text{s)}}{\text{medium one propagation speed (mm/}\mu\text{s)}}\right]$	$\Theta_t = \Theta_i \left[\dfrac{c_2}{c_1}\right]$

The second equation is called **Snell's law.** A change in direction of sound when crossing a boundary is called **refraction** (Latin: to turn aside). The transmission angle is greater than the incidence angle if the propagation speed through medium two is greater than the propagation speed through medium one [Figure 3.4(a)]. There is no refraction if the propagation speeds are equal [Figure 3.4(b)] or if the incidence angle is zero (perpendicular incidence).

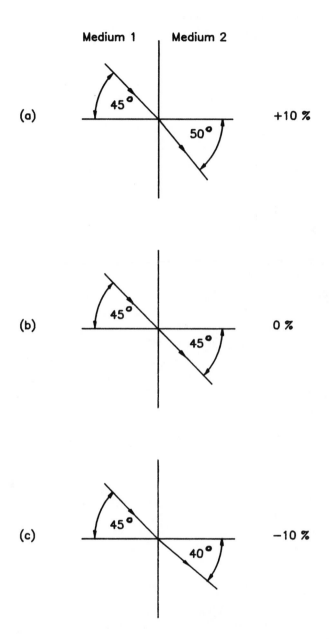

Figure 3.4. Transmission angles for an incidence angle of 45 degrees and propagation speeds through medium two (a) 10 percent greater than, (b) equal to, and (c) 10 percent less than propagation speed through medium one.

Example If the incidence angle is 20 degrees, the propagation speed in medium
3.3.1. one is 1600 m/s, and the propagation speed in medium two is 1400
m/s, calculate the reflection and transmission angles.

$$\text{reflection angle} = \text{incidence angle} = 20°$$

$$\text{transmission angle} = \text{incidence angle} \times \left[\frac{\text{speed}_2}{\text{speed}_1}\right]$$

$$= 20\left(\frac{1400}{1600}\right) = 17.5°$$

Refraction occurs with light as well as with sound. It is the principle
on which lenses operate. It is also the cause of distortion when viewing
objects in a fish bowl. As with sound, when light crosses a boundary
obliquely, where a change in light speed occurs, the direction of the
light travel changes.

Expressions for calculating reflection and transmission coefficients
are more complicated than those that apply when there is perpendicular
incidence, and they are not given here. For given media, the reflection
coefficient for oblique incidence may be smaller than, equal to, or
greater than that for normal incidence, depending on incidence angle.
If the propagation speeds through the media are the same, the intensity
reflection coefficient is the same as that for perpendicular incidence
(see Section 3.2) and is independent of incidence angle. For oblique
incidence it is possible for a reflection to occur even if the media have
equal impedances. This will occur if the propagation speeds are different. Conversely, it is possible that no reflection will occur even when
the media impedances are different. Therefore, absence of reflection
with oblique incidence does not necessarily mean that the media
impedances are equal (as it did with perpendicular incidence).

Exercises

3.3.1. Refraction is a change in _____ of sound
when it crosses a boundary.

3.3.2. If the propagation speed through medium two is larger than
the propagation speed through medium one, the
transmission angle will be _____
_____the incidence angle, and the
reflection angle will be _____
_____ the incidence angle.

3.3.3. If the propagation speed through medium two is smaller than the propagation speed through medium one, the transmission angle will be _____ _____ the incidence angle, and the reflection angle will be _____ _____ the incidence angle.

3.3.4. If the propagation speed through medium two is equal to the propagation speed through medium one, the transmission angle will be _____ _____ the incidence angle, and the reflection angle will be _____ _____ the incidence angle.

3.3.5. If the incidence angle is 30 degrees, the propagation speed through medium one is 1000 m/s, and the propagation speed through medium two is 700 m/s, the reflection angle is _____ degrees and the transmission angle is _____ degrees.

3.3.6. If the incidence angle is 30 degrees, the propagation speed through medium one is 1000 m/s, and the propagation speed through medium two is 1000 m/s, the reflection angle is _____ degrees and the transmission angle is _____ degrees.

3.3.7. If the incidence angle is 30 degrees and the propagation speed through medium two is 30 percent higher than the propagation speed through medium one, the reflection angle is _____ degrees and the transmission angle is _____ degrees.

3.3.8. Given the following:
incidence angle = 20 degrees
incident intensity = 5 mW/cm^2
propagation speed through medium one = 1500 m/s
impedance of medium one = 8 rayls
propagation speed through medium two = 1500 m/s
impedance of medium two = 12 rayls,
the reflection coefficient is _____ .

3.3.9. Given the following:
incidence angle = 20 degrees
incident intensity = 5 mW/cm^2
transmission angle = 20 degrees
impedance of medium one = 8 rayls
impedance of medium two = 12 rayls,
the reflected intensity is _____ mW/cm^2.

3.3.10. Under what two conditions does refraction not occur?
a. _____
b. _____

3.3.11. Under what condition is the reflection coefficient not dependent on incidence angle?

_____

3.3.12. When ultrasound encounters a boundary with oblique incidence, either _____ or _____ _____ must change in order to generate a reflection.

3.3.13. The low speed of sound in fat is a source of image degradation because of refraction. If the incidence angle at a boundary between fat (1440 m/s) and kidney (1560 m/s) is 30 degrees, the transmission angle is _____ degrees.

3.3.14. For Problem 3.3.13, the lateral shift of the sound path 5 cm beyond the boundary because of refraction is _____ mm. Proceed as follows: The difference between the incidence and transmission angles is 2 degrees. The tangent of 2 degrees is .0349. The tangent multiplied by the distance (5 cm) yields the lateral shift.

3.4
Scattering

In Sections 3.2 and 3.3 it was assumed that wavelength is small compared with the boundary dimensions and with boundary roughness. The resulting reflections are called **specular reflections**. If, on the other hand, the boundary dimensions are comparable to or small compared with the wavelength, or if the boundary is not smooth (surface irregularities comparable in size to the wavelength), the incident sound will be scattered (diffused). Scattering is the redirection of sound in many directions by rough surfaces or by heterogeneous media such as (cellular) tissues or particle suspensions such as blood (Figure 3.5). These cases are analogous to light in which specular (Latin: mirror) reflections occur at mirrors. For a rougher surface, such as a white wall, although virtually all the light is reflected (that is why the wall is white) the image is not observed (as in a mirror) because the light is scattered at the surface and mixed up as it travels back to the viewer's eyes. When light passes through a suspension of water droplets in air (fog) it is scattered as well. This limits the viewer's ability to see through fog. Although scattering inhibits vision (we cannot see ourselves reflected in a wall and we cannot see well through fog), it is of great benefit in ultrasound imaging. Here the desire is to see the "wall" (tissue interface), not a reflection of "oneself" (the sound source). There is also a desire to see the "fog" (tissue parenchyma), not just objects beyond it.

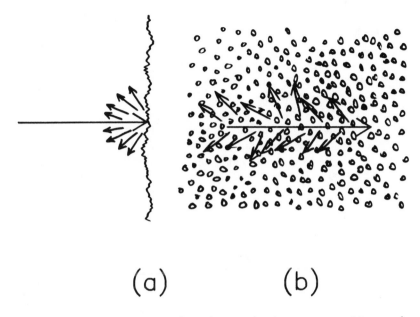

$$(a) \qquad (b)$$

Figure 3.5. Scattering occurs when ultrasound pulses encounter (a) a rough surface or (b) a heterogeneous medium, such as tissue.

Backscatter (sound scattered back in the direction from which it originally came) intensities from rough surfaces and heterogeneous media vary with frequency and scatterer size. They may be comparable to or less than specular reflection intensities from tissue boundaries. Normally, scatter intensities are much less than boundary specular reflection intensities. The roughness of a tissue boundary or heterogeneity of a medium (such as tissue) effectively increases as frequency is increased (increased backscatter). This is because wavelength decreases as frequency increases, thus making wavelength smaller relative to roughness or scatterer dimensions. This is why the sky is blue. Light is more strongly scattered by particles suspended in the atmosphere for higher frequencies (low frequency light is red, high frequency light is blue).

The intensity received by the sound source from specular reflections is highly angle-dependent (see Figure 8.5). Scattering from boundaries helps to make echo reception less dependent on incidence angle.

Scattering, then, permits ultrasound imaging of tissue boundaries that are not necessarily perpendicular to the direction of the incident sound. It also allows imaging of tissue parenchyma as well as organ boundaries. Scattering is relatively independent of the direction of the incident sound and therefore is more characteristic of the scatterers.

Reflections from smooth boundaries depend not only on the acoustic properties at the boundaries but also on the angles involved.

Since the ultrasound pulse encounters several scatterers at any point in its travel, several echoes are generated simultaneously. These may arrive at the transducer in such a way that they reinforce (constructive interference) or partially or totally cancel (destructive interference) each other. This results in a displayed dot pattern that does not directly represent scatterers, but rather an interference pattern of the scatterer distribution scanned. This phenomenon is called acoustic **speckle**. It is analagous to the speckle phenomenon observed with lasers.

Exercises

3.4.1. Redirection of sound in many directions as it encounters rough media junctions or particle suspensions (heterogeneous media) is called _____ .

3.4.2. With specular reflection, wavelength is small compared with boundary dimensions. True or false?

3.4.3. Scattering occurs when boundary dimensions are large compared with wavelength or when the boundary is smooth. True or false?

3.4.4. As frequency increases, backscatter strength
a. increases
b. decreases
c. does not change
d. refracts
e. infarcts

3.4.5. Backscatter helps make echo reception less dependent on incidence angle. True or false?

3.4.6. As frequency increases, specular reflections
a. increase
b. decrease
c. do not change
d. refract
e. infarct

3.5 Range Equation

Now that sound propagation, reflection, and scattering have been considered, a very important factor for **pulse-echo diagnostic ultrasound,** the **range equation**, can be studied. The approach in pulse-echo diagnostic ultrasound is (1) to generate short pulses of sound that travel through the body, producing reflections **(echoes)** that travel back

to the source and (2) to detect and display the returning echoes. The
method that the instrumentation uses to properly position the echo on
the display will be described in Chapter 5. The two items of information
required are (1) the direction from which the echo came (which is
assumed to be the direction in which the source is pointed) and (2)
the distance to the boundary (**reflector** or **scatterer**) where the echo
was produced. The distance is calculated from the range (distance-to-
reflector) equation:

distance to reflector (mm) = ½ [propagation speed (mm/μs) × pulse round-trip time (μs)]	$d = \frac{1}{2} ct$

To get the distance from the source to the reflector, the propagation
speed in the intervening medium must be known or assumed, and the
pulse round-trip time must be measured. The reason that the factor ½
appears is that the round-trip time is the time for the pulse to travel to
the reflector and return; only the distance *to* the reflector is desired.
The soft-tissue average propagation speed (1.54 mm/μs) is usually assumed in using the range equation (unless another speed is given). For
this case:

For soft tissues: distance to reflector (mm) $\overset{*}{=}$ 0.77 × pulse round-trip time (μs)	$d \overset{*}{=} 0.77t$

The previous equation was derived from the range equation by substituting 1.54 for the speed and dividing by 2 to get 0.77.

Exercises

3.5.1. The approach in pulse-echo ultrasound is (1) to generate
_____ of sound that travel through the
body, producing _____ that travel back
to the source, and (2) to detect and
_____ the returning echoes.

3.5.2. To calculate the distance to a reflector, the
_____ _____ and the
pulse round-trip _____ must be known.

3.5.3. If the propagation speed is 1.6 mm/μs and the pulse round-
trip time is 5 μs, the distance to the reflector is _____ mm.

3.5.4. If the propagation speed is 1.4 mm/μs and the time for a
pulse to travel to the reflector is 5 μs, the distance to the
reflector is _____ mm.

3.5.5. When the pulse round-trip time is 10 μs, the distance to a reflector in soft tissue is _____ mm.

3.5.6. When the pulse round-trip time is 13 μs, the distance to a reflector in soft tissue is _____ cm.

**3.6
Review**
When sound encounters (with *perpendicular incidence*) boundaries between media with different impedances, part of the sound is reflected and part is transmitted. If the two media have the same impedance, there is no reflection. With *oblique incidence*, the sound is refracted at a boundary between media where propagation speeds are different. Incidence and reflection angles are always equal. For oblique incidence there may be a reflection when the impedances are equal (if the propagation speeds are different), and there may not be a reflection even if the impedances are different. Scattering occurs at rough media boundaries and within heterogeneous media. The range equation is used to determine distance to reflectors.

Exercises

3.6.1. If no refraction occurs as an oblique sound beam passes through the boundary between two materials, the _____ _____ of the materials are known to be _____ .

3.6.2. What must be known in order to calculate distance to a reflector?
a. attenuation, speed, density
b. attenuation, impedance
c. attenuation, absorption
d. travel time, speed
e. density, speed

3.6.3. With perpendicular incidence, if the impedances of two media are the same, there will be no
a. inflation
b. reflection
c. refraction
d. calibration
e. both b and c

3.6.4. What is the transmitted intensity if the incident intensity is 1 and the impedances are 1.00 and 2.64?
a. 0.2
b. 0.4
c. 0.6
d. 0.8
e. 1.0

3.6.5. If the incident intensity is 1 and the impedances are 3 and 2, the reflected intensity is _____ .

3.6.6. No reflection will occur with perpendicular incidence if the media _____ are equal.

3.6.7. No reflection will occur with oblique incidence if the media _____ are equal and the media _____ _____ are equal.

3.6.8. If the incidence angle is 20 degrees and the propagation speeds of media one and two are 1700 and 1500, respectively, the transmission angle is _____ degrees.

3.6.9. If the incidence angle is 20 degrees and propagation speeds of media one and two are 1500 and 1700, respectively, the transmission angle is _____ degrees.

3.6.10. Scattering occurs at smooth boundaries and within homogeneous media. True or false?

Chapter 4

Transducers and Sound Beams

**4.1
Introduction**

The characteristics of ultrasound that are important for diagnosis have been described in Chapters 2 and 3. In this chapter the devices that generate and receive ultrasound will be described. They form the connecting link (see Figure 1.2) between the ultrasound/tissue interactions of Figure 1.1 and the instrumentation described in Chapters 5–7. Except for mention of sound beams in Section 2.4, the confining of sound to beams has not yet been covered. The devices described in this chapter do not produce sound that travels uniformly in all directions away from the source; rather, the sound is confined in beams, which will be described in Section 4.3. Transducers specific to dynamic imaging instruments are described in Chapter 6.

**4.2
Transducers**

Transducers convert one form of energy to another (see Appendix D). Examples are given in Table 4.1. **Ultrasound transducers** have no special name such as microphone or loudspeaker, which are the names applied to devices that accomplish similar functions with audible sound. Ultrasound transducers convert electrical energy into ultrasound energy and vice versa. **Electric voltages** applied to them are converted to ultrasound. Ultrasound incident on them produces electric voltages.

Table 4.1

Transducer Examples

Transducer	converts	to
Light bulb	electricity	light and heat
Automobile engine	chemical energy	motion and heat
Ear	sound	nerve impulses
Oven	electricity	heat
Motor	electricity	motion
Generator	motion	electricity
Battery	chemical energy	electricity
Human	chemical energy	heat, motion, and sound
Microphone	audible sound	electricity
Loudspeaker	electricity	audible sound

Ultrasound transducers operate on the **piezoelectricity** (from Greek: pressure-electricity) principle, which was discovered in 1880. The principle states that some materials (ceramics, quartz, and others) produce a voltage when deformed by an applied pressure. Piezoelectricity also results in production of a pressure when these materials are deformed by an applied voltage. The materials most commonly used in diagnostic ultrasound transducers are mixtures of lead zirconate and lead titanate. Ceramics such as these are not *naturally* piezoelectric. They are made piezoelectric during production by placing them in a strong electric field while they are at high temperature.

Single-element transducers (other types are discussed in Chapter 6) are in the form of **discs** (Figure 4.1). When an electric voltage is applied to the faces, the thickness of the disc increases or decreases depending on the polarity of the voltage. The term **transducer element** (also called piezoelectric element or active element) refers to the piece of piezoelectric material that converts electricity to ultrasound and vice versa. The element with its associated case and damping and matching materials (discussed later in this section) is called the **transducer assembly** or **probe** (Figure 4.2). Both the transducer element and the transducer assembly are commonly referred to as the transducer. Typical diagnostic ultrasound transducer elements are 6 to 19 mm in diameter and 0.2 to 2 mm thick.

Source transducers operated in the **continuous mode (continuous wave mode)** are driven by a continuous alternating voltage (see Chapter 7) and produce an alternating pressure that propagates as a sound wave [Figure 4.3(a)]. The frequency of the sound produced is equal to the frequency of the driving voltage. The operating frequency (sometimes

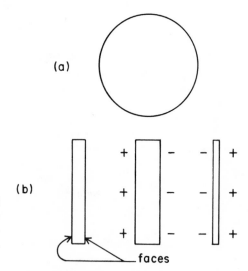

(a)

(b)

faces

Figure 4.1. A disc transducer element. (a) Front view. (b) Side view with no voltage applied to faces (normal thickness), voltage applied (increased thickness), and voltage of opposite polarity applied (decreased thickness).

called **resonance frequency**) of the transducer is its preferred frequency of operation. Operating frequency is determined by the propagation speed of the transducer material (typically 4–6 mm/μs) and the thickness of the transducer element.

$$\text{operating frequency (MHz)} = \frac{\text{propagation speed (mm/μs)}}{2 \times \text{thickness (mm)}} \qquad f_o = \frac{c_m}{2w}$$

where propagation speed is that for the transducer material.

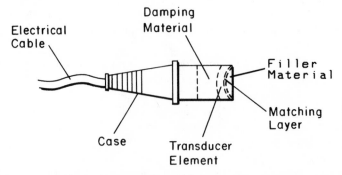

Figure 4.2. A transducer assembly or probe. The damping material reduces pulse duration, thus improving axial resolution. The matching layer increases sound transmission into the tissues. The filler material enables the face of the transducer assembly to be flat. The transducer element is usually curved for focusing (Section 4.3), but is sometimes flat (unfocused).

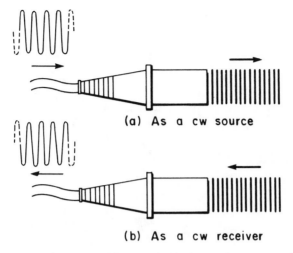

Figure 4.3. A transducer assembly operating in the continuous wave (cw) mode. The device converts (a) a cw voltage into cw ultrasound or converts (b) received cw ultrasound into a cw voltage.

Continuous-wave sound encountering a receiving transducer is converted to a continuous alternating voltage [Figure 4.3(b)]. For instruments employing the continuous-wave mode, separate source and receiver transducer elements are required, since they each must continuously perform their function. These elements are built into a single transducer assembly.

Source transducers operated in the **pulsed mode** (pulsed ultrasound) are driven by **voltage pulses** (see Section 5.2) and produce ultrasound pulses (Figure 4.4). These transducers convert received reflections into voltage pulses. The pulse repetition frequency is equal to the voltage pulse repetition frequency, which is determined by the instrument driving the transducer. The pulse duration is equal to the period (reciprocal of operating frequency) multiplied by the number of cycles in the pulse (see Section 2.3). Damping material (a mixture of metal powder and a plastic or epoxy) is attached to the rear face of the transducer element to reduce the number of cycles in each pulse (Figure 4.5). This reduces pulse duration and spatial pulse length and thus results in improved axial resolution (Section 4.4). This method of damping is analogous to packing foam rubber around a bell that is rung by a tap with a hammer. The rubber reduces the time that the bell rings following the tap. It also reduces the loudness or intensity of the ringing. For ultrasound transducers, the damping material reduces the ultrasound amplitude and thus decreases the efficiency and **sensitivity** of the system (undesired effect). This is the price paid for reduced spatial pulse length (desired effect resulting in improved axial reso-

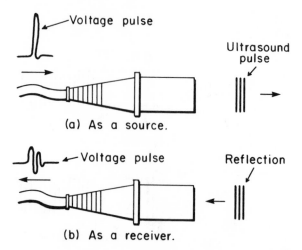

Figure 4.4. A transducer assembly operating in the pulsed mode. This device converts (a) electric voltage pulses into ultrasound pulses and converts (b) received ultrasound pulses (reflections) into electric voltage pulses.

lution). Some damping may also be accomplished electrically within the instrument. Typically, pulses of two or three cycles are generated with diagnostic ultrasound transducers.

A **matching layer** is commonly placed on the transducer face (see Figure 4.2). This material has an impedance intermediate between those of the transducer element and the tissue. It reduces the reflection of ultrasound at the transducer element surface, improving sound transmission across it. This is analogous to the coating layer on a camera lens, which reduces light reflection at the air–glass boundary. The optimum thickness for this matching layer is one quarter of a wavelength. Because many frequencies and wavelengths are present in short ultrasound pulses (see below), multiple matching layers provide a greater improvement in sound transmission across the element–tissue boundary.

Because of its very low impedance, even a very thin layer of air between the transducer and the skin surface will reflect virtually all the sound, preventing any penetration into the tissue. For this reason, a coupling medium, usually an aqueous gel or mineral oil, is applied to the skin before transducer contact. This eliminates the air layer and permits the sound to pass into the tissue.

A transducer operating in the pulsed mode prefers to produce a frequency equal to its operating frequency (introduced earlier in this section). However, the ultrasound pulses produced contain frequencies in addition to this. The shorter the pulse (the fewer the number of cycles), the more frequencies that are present. The range of frequencies

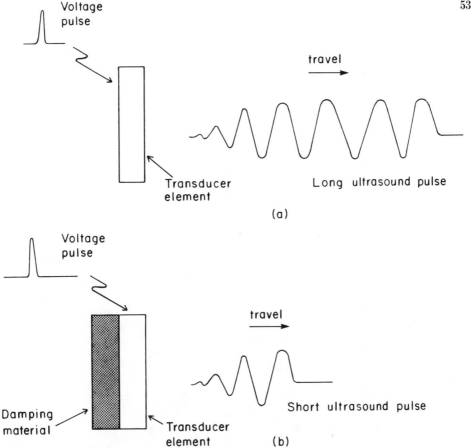

Figure 4.5. Without damping (a), a voltage pulse applied to a transducer element results in a long pulse of many cycles. With damping material on the rear face of the transducer element (b), application of a voltage pulse results in a short pulse of a few cycles. This figure shows each pulse traveling away from the transducer from left to right in space so that the right-hand end is the beginning or leading edge of the pulse.

involved in a pulse is called its **bandwidth** (Figure 4.6). **Fractional bandwidth** is equal to the bandwidth divided by the operating frequency. **Quality factor** (Q factor) is equal to operating frequency divided by the bandwidth, that is the reciprocal of the fractional bandwidth:

$$\text{quality factor} = \frac{\text{operating frequency (MHz)}}{\text{bandwidth (MHz)}} \qquad Q = \frac{f_o}{BW}$$

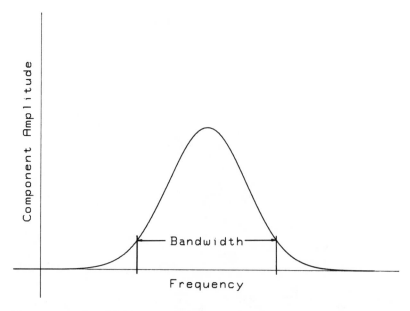

Figure 4.6. A plot of the frequencies present in an ultrasound pulse. Component amplitude is the amplitude of each frequency component present. Bandwidth is the frequency range within which the amplitudes exceed some reference value.

Quality factor is unitless. The inclusion of damping material in the transducer assembly increases the bandwidth and decreases the quality factor. For short (2 or 3 cycle) pulses, the quality factor is approximately equal to the number of cycles in the pulse. The overall *system* bandwidth is determined not only by the transducer but also by the instrument electronics.

Exercises

4.2.1. A transducer converts one form of _____ to another.

4.2.2. Ultrasound transducers convert _____ energy into _____ energy and vice versa.

4.2.3. Ultrasound transducers operate on the _____ principle.

4.2.4. Single-element transducers are in the form of _____ .

4.2.5. The _____ of a transducer element changes when a voltage is applied to the faces.

4.2.6. The term transducer is often used to refer to either a transducer _____ or a transducer _____ .

4.2.7. A transducer _____ is part of a transducer _____ .

4.2.8. A continuously alternating voltage applied to a transducer produces _____ ultrasound.

4.2.9. Electrical voltage pulses applied to a transducer produce ultrasound _____ .

4.2.10. Operating frequency _____ as transducer element thickness is increased.

4.2.11. Addition of damping material to a transducer reduces the number of _____ in the pulse, thus improving _____ _____ . It increases the _____ and decreases the _____ _____ .

4.2.12. Addition of damping material reduces the _____ and _____ of the diagnostic system.

4.2.13. Ultrasound transducers typically generate pulses of _____ or _____ cycles.

4.2.14. If the propagation speed of the transducer element material is 4 mm/μs, the thickness required for an operating frequency of 10 MHz is _____ mm.

4.2.15. If the propagation speed of the transducer element material is 6 mm/μs, the operating frequency for a thickness of 0.2 mm is _____ MHz.

4.2.16. The matching layer on the transducer surface reduces _____ caused by impedance difference.

4.2.17. A coupling medium on the skin surface eliminates reflection caused by _____ .

4.2.18. Quality factor is given in
a. MHz
b. mm/μs
c. percent
d. all of the above
e. none of the above

4.2.19. Increasing the bandwidth increases the quality factor. True or false?

4.2.20. The range of _____ involved in an ultrasound pulse is called its bandwidth.

4.2.21. A two-cycle pulse has a Q factor of approximately _____ .
a. 0.2
b. 0.5
c. 2
d. 5
e. 20

4.2.22. If bandwidth is 1 MHz and operating frequency is 3 MHz calculate the following:
a. Q factor _____
b. fractional bandwidth _____
c. lowest frequency _____
d. highest frequency _____
e. approximate number of cycles per pulse _____

**4.3
Beams
and
Focusing**

The ultrasound pulse generated by the (flat) disc transducer in Figure 4.1 is contained in a cylindrical shape, as shown in Figure 4.7. The spatial pulse length was discussed in Sections 2.3 and 4.2. This section is concerned with the pulse diameter. The sound beam is a description of this diameter as the pulse travels away from the transducer.

A single-element (flat) disc transducer operating in the continuous-wave mode produces a sound beam with a beam diameter that varies according to the distance from the transducer face as shown in Figure 4.8. The intensity is not uniform throughout the beam (Section 2.4). The beam diameter shown in Figure 4.8 approximates that portion of the sound produced that is greater than 4 percent of the spatial peak intensity. This particular value was chosen because it gives the simplest picture. The 6-dB beam diameter that is often used is narrower than that pictured in Figure 4.8. It includes that portion of the sound that is greater than 25 percent of the spatial peak intensity. Sometimes significant intensity travels out in some directions not included in the beam as pictured. These additional "beams" are called **side lobes**.

The region from the disc out to a distance of one near-zone length is called the **near zone**, near field, or Fresnel zone. Near-zone length (also called near-field length) is given by the equations:

$$\text{near-zone length (mm)} = \frac{[\text{transducer diameter (mm)}]^2}{4 \times \text{wavelength (mm)}} \qquad \text{NZL} = \frac{D_T^2}{4\lambda}$$

For soft tissues:
$$\text{near-zone length (mm)} \stackrel{*}{=} \frac{[\text{transducer diameter (mm)}]^2 \times \text{frequency (MHz)}}{6} \qquad \text{NZL} \stackrel{*}{=} \frac{D_T^2 f}{6}$$

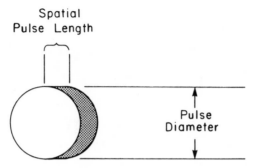

Spatial
Pulse Length

Pulse
Diameter

Figure 4.7. An ultrasound pulse generated by a single-element disc transducer driven by an electric voltage pulse as shown in Figure 4.4. The pulse diameter is equal to beam diameter. This varies with distance from the transducer (Figure 4.8). Spatial pulse length is described in Figure 2.8.

The second equation is derived from the first by substituting for wavelength, propagation speed (1.54 mm/μs for soft tissues) divided by frequency. Table 4.2 lists near-zone lengths for various transducer frequencies and diameters.

The region beyond a distance of one near-zone length is called the **far zone**, far field, or Fraunhofer zone.

The beam diameter depends on

1. wavelength (therefore frequency)
2. transducer diameter
3. distance from transducer

In the approximation of Figure 4.8, at a distance of one near-zone length from the transducer, the beam diameter is equal to one-half the transducer diameter. At a distance of two times the near-zone length, the beam diameter is equal to the transducer diameter. Beyond this distance, the beam diameter increases in proportion to distance.

The diameter of an ultrasound pulse (Figure 4.7) is equal to the beam diameter (Figure 4.8) for the distance from the transducer face at which the pulse is located at any given time. As the pulse travels through the near zone, its diameter decreases; as it travels through the far zone, its diameter increases.

Sound beams produced by disc transducers have beam areas given by the equation:

beam area (cm²) = 0.8 × [beam diameter (cm)]²	$A_B = 0.8\ D_B^2$

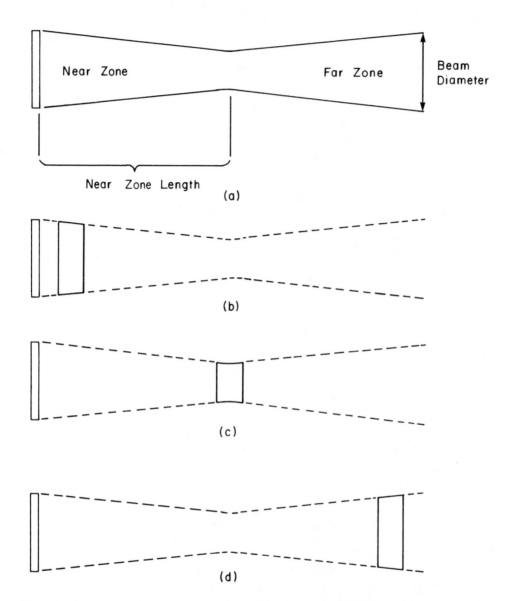

Figure 4.8. Beam diameter for a single-element unfocused disc transducer operating in the continuous-wave mode (a). This diameter approximates the region of that portion of the sound produced that is greater than 4 percent of the spatial peak intensity. The near zone is the region between the disc and the minimum beam diameter. The far zone is the region beyond the minimum beam diameter. Intensity is not constant within the beam. Intensity variations are greatest in the near zone. The beam diameter in (a) approximates the changing pulse diameter as an ultrasound pulse travels away from the transducer. (b) A pulse shortly after leaving the transducer. (c) Later the pulse is located at the near-zone length, where its diameter is a minimum. (d) Later the pulse is in the far field, where its diameter is increasing as it travels. This figure assumes a nonscattering nonrefracting medium such as water.

Table 4.2
Near-zone Length (NZL) for Unfocused Transducers

Frequency (MHz)	Diameter (mm)	NZL (cm)
2.25	19	13
3.5	13	10
3.5	19	20
5.0	6	3
5.0	10	8
5.0	13	14
7.5	6	4
10.0	6	6

For soft tissue and a 10-mm 5-MHz transducer, what are the beam diameters 8 and 16 cm from the transducer? First find the near-zone length:

Example 4.3.1

$$\text{near-zone length} = \frac{(\text{transducer diameter})^2 \times \text{frequency}}{6}$$

$$\frac{10^2 \times 5}{6} = 83 \text{ mm} = 8.3 \text{ cm}$$

A distance of 8 cm is therefore near the end of the near zone. The beam diameter is therefore approximately equal to one half the transducer element diameter, i.e., 5 mm. A distance of 16 cm is in the far zone at approximately double the near-zone length. Therefore, the beam diameter at this point is approximately equal to the transducer element diameter, 10 mm.

The effects of frequency on near-zone length and beam diameter are shown in Figure 4.9 The effects of transducer diameter are shown in Figure 4.10 The beam dimensions for those figures are calculated in Problems 4.3.11 through 4.3.18.

An increase in frequency or transducer size increases the near-zone length. When sufficiently far from the transducer, increasing frequency or the transducer size can *decrease* the beam diameter (Figures 4.9 and 4.10).

For improved **lateral resolution** (Section 4.4), beam diameter is reduced by focusing the sound in a manner similar to the focusing of light. Sound may be focused (Figure 4.11) by employing a curved (rather than a flat) transducer element, a curved reflector in the transducer assembly, a lens, or a phased **array** (see Chapter 6). **"Internal focus"** refers to the use of a curved transducer element. Beam diameter is decreased in the **focal region** and between it and the transducer; it is widened in the region beyond (Figure 4.12). **Focal length** is the distance

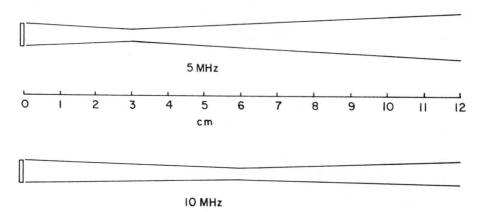

5 MHz

0　1　2　3　4　5　6　7　8　9　10　11　12

cm

10 MHz

Figure 4.9. Beams for 6-mm diameter disc transducers of two frequencies. Higher frequency produces smaller beam diameter (beyond 4 cm) and longer near-zone length.

from the transducer to the center of the focal region or to the location of the spatial peak intensity. Manufacturers use qualitative terms such as short, medium, or long internal focus to indicate the length of focal regions or focal length. The two normally go together, i.e., long focal lengths are associated with long focal regions. Numerical values associated with these terms vary with manufacturers. The focal length cannot be greater than the near-zone length of the comparable (same transducer diameter and operating frequency) unfocused transducers. Focal zone is specified as the distance between two points at the center of the beam at which the intensity is some fraction (commonly 25 percent, 6 dB) of the peak intensity at the focus. A second way of

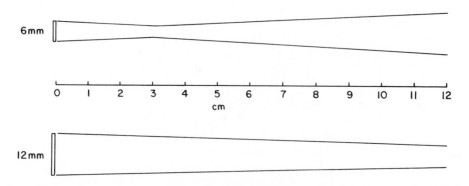

6mm

0　1　2　3　4　5　6　7　8　9　10　11　12

cm

12mm

Figure 4.10. Beams for 5-MHz disc transducers of two diameters. The larger transducer produces the larger near-zone length. The right-hand portion of the figure shows that a smaller transducer can produce a larger-diameter beam. The beam diameters are equal at a distance of 8 cm.

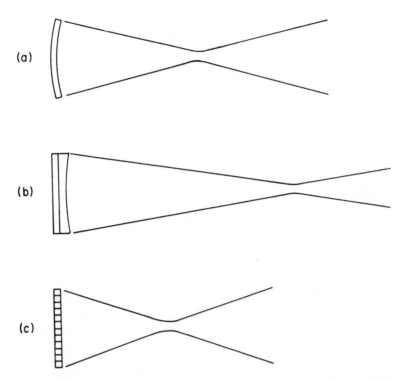

Figure 4.11. Sound focusing by (a) a curved transducer, (b) a lens, and (c) a phased array. Lenses focus because the propagation speed through them is higher than that through tissues. Refraction (see Section 3.3) at the surface of the lens forms the beam such that a focal region occurs. The operation of phased arrays is described in Section 6.2. The amount by which the beam diameter is reduced by focusing is described qualitatively as weak or strong focus.

specifying focal zone is the distance between equal beam widths or diameters that are some multiple (e.g., two times) of the minimum value (at the focus). Most diagnostic imaging transducers are focused to some degree.

Exercises

4.3.1. The beam diameter in Figure 4.8 includes that portion of the sound produced that is greater than _____ percent of the spatial peak intensity.

4.3.2. The beam is divided into two regions called the _____ zone and the _____ zone.

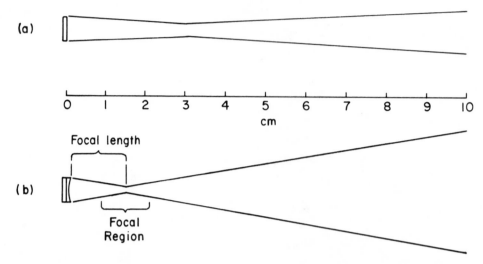

Figure 4.12. Beam diameter for 6-mm 5-MHz disc transducer of Figures 4.9 and 4.10 without (a) and with (b) a focusing lens. Focusing in this case produces a minimum beam diameter half that for nonfocusing. However, beyond 2.5 cm from the transducer (outside the focal region), the focused beam diameter is greater than the unfocused.

4.3.3. The dividing point between the two regions is at a distance from the transducer equal to one _____ length.

4.3.4. Beam diameter depends on _____, transducer _____ , and _____ from the transducer.

4.3.5. Near-zone length is proportional to the square of the _____ and inversely proportional to _____ .

4.3.6. For a given medium (a given propagation speed), near-zone length is proportional to the square of the _____ _____ and to the _____ .

4.3.7. At a distance of one near-zone length from the transducer, beam diameter is equal to _____ transducer diameter.

4.3.8. At a distance of _____ times the near-zone length, beam diameter is equal to transducer diameter.

4.3.9. In the near zone, beam diameter _____ as distance from the transducer increases.

4.3.10. In the far zone, beam diameter _____ as distance from the transducer increases.

4.3.11. For soft tissue and a 6-mm 5-MHz transducer (Figures 4.9 and 4.10), the near-zone length is _____ mm.

4.3.12. For Problem 4.3.11, the beam diameters at 15, 30, 60 and 120 mm from the transducer are _____ , _____, _____and _____ mm, respectively.

4.3.13. For soft tissue and a 6-mm 10-MHz transducer (Figure 4.9), the near-zone length is _____ mm.

4.3.14. For Problem 4.3.13, the beam diameters at 60, 120, and 180 mm from the transducer are _____ , _____ , and _____ mm, respectively.

4.3.15. In Problems 4.3.11 to 4.3.14, the higher-frequency transducer produces the _____ near-zone length and the _____ beam diameter at 60 mm from the transducer.

4.3.16. For soft tissue and a 12-mm 5-MHz transducer (Figure 4.10), the near-zone length is _____ mm.

4.3.17. For Problem 4.3.16, the beam diameters at 60, 120, 180, and 240 mm from the transducer are _____ , _____ , _____ , and _____ mm, respectively.

4.3.18. In Problems 4.3.11, 4.3.12, 4.3.16, and 4.3.17, the larger transducer produces the _____ near-zone length and the _____ beam diameter at 120 mm from the transducer.

4.3.19. Doubling the transducer diameter _____ the near-zone length.

4.3.20. Doubling the frequency _____ the near-zone length.

4.3.21. If transducer diameter is doubled and frequency is halved, the near-zone length is _____ .

4.3.22. Sound may be focused by employing a
a. curved element
b. curved reflector
c. lense
d. phased array
e. more than one of the above

4.3.23. Focusing reduces the beam diameter at all distances from the transducer. True or false?

4.3.24. _____ _____ is the distance from the transducer to the location of the spatial peak intensity produced by a focused transducer.

4.4 Resolution and Useful Frequency Range

If two reflectors are not sufficiently separated, they will not produce separate reflections and thus will not be separated on the instrumentation display. Characteristics of the instrumentation electronics and display may further degrade this acoustic resolution. It is apparent, however, that if separate reflections are not initially generated the reflectors will not be separated on the display. In ultrasound imaging there are two aspects to resolution: **axial** and lateral. They depend on different characteristics of the ultrasound pulses as they travel through the tissues.

The important parameter in determining the required separation for resolution along the direction of the sound travel (axial resolution) is the spatial pulse length (Section 2.3). The axial resolution is the minimum reflector separation required along the direction of sound travel so that separate reflections will be produced (Figure 4.13). It is also called longitudinal, range, or depth resolution.

$\text{axial resolution (mm)} = \dfrac{\text{spatial pulse length (mm)}}{2}$ For soft tissues: $\text{axial resolution (mm)} \overset{*}{=} \dfrac{0.77 \times \text{number of cycles in the pulse}}{\text{frequency (MHz)}}$	$R_A = \dfrac{SPL}{2}$ $R_A = \dfrac{0.77n}{f}$

The second equation is derived from the first by substituting for spatial pulse length according to the last equation in the box on page 15.

Axial resolution is like a golf score—the smaller the better. The smaller it is, the more detail that can be displayed and the closer two reflectors can be along the sound path and still be seen distinctly. To improve axial resolution, spatial pulse length must be reduced. Since spatial pulse length is the product of wavelength and the number of cycles in the pulse (see Section 2.3), one or both of these must be reduced. For a given propagation speed (such as 1.54 mm/μs in soft tissue), wavelength is reduced as frequency is increased (see Section 2.2). The number of cycles in each pulse may be reduced by increasing transducer **damping;** this was discussed in Section 4.2. If the number of cycles per pulse is reduced to a minimum (2 or 3), the only way to further improve axial resolution is to increase frequency:

> Axial resolution improves as frequency increases.

When this is done, however, there is a price to be paid. It is a reduction in half-intensity depth (Section 2.5), because attenuation increases as frequency increases:

> Half-intensity depth decreases as frequency increases.

In order to reasonably meet resolution and imaging depth requirements, the useful frequency range is restricted to between 1 and 10 MHz. The lower portion of the range is useful where large depth (e.g., an obese subject) or high attenuation is encountered. The higher portion of the frequency range is useful where small depth is required (e.g., in imaging the breast, eye, thyroid, or superficial vessels or in pediatric imaging). In most large patients, 3.5 MHz is a satisfactory frequency, while in thin patients and children, 5 and 7.5 MHz can often be used. If frequencies less than 1 MHz are used, the axial resolution is not sufficient. If frequencies higher than 10 MHz (less than 10 MHz in many applications) are used, the depth is not sufficient.

Table 4.3 gives values for half-intensity depth (from Table 2.6) and (two-cycle pulse) axial resolution for various frequencies. Half-intensity depth in millimeters is equal to 30 divided by frequency in megahertz. Axial resolution in millimeters for a two-cycle pulse in soft tissue is equal to 1.54 divided by frequency in megahertz. Therefore, for a two-cycle pulse in soft tissue, half-intensity depth is approximately 20 times axial resolution.

Lateral resolution is the minimum separation (in the direction perpendicular to the direction of sound travel or the direction of the beam) between two reflectors such that when the beam is scanned across them, two separate reflections are produced (Figure 4.14). Lateral resolution is equal to beam diameter.

lateral resolution (mm) = beam diameter (mm)	$R_l = D_B$

Recall that beam diameter varies with distance from the transducer, and therefore so does lateral resolution. If the lateral separation between two reflectors is greater than the beam diameter, two separate reflections are produced when the beam is scanned across them. Thus they are resolved, i.e., detected as separate reflectors.

Lateral resolution is also called transverse, angular, and azimuthal resolution. As with axial resolution, a smaller value indicates an improvement (finer detail is imaged). Lateral resolution may be improved by reducing the beam diameter. This may be done by increasing the

Table 4.3
Half-intensity Depth and Axial Resolution (Two-Cycle Pulse) in Tissue

Frequency (MHz)	Half-intensity Depth (mm)	Axial Resolution (mm)
1.00	30	1.5
2.25	13	0.7
3.50	9	0.4
5.00	6	0.3
7.50	4	0.2
10.00	3	0.2

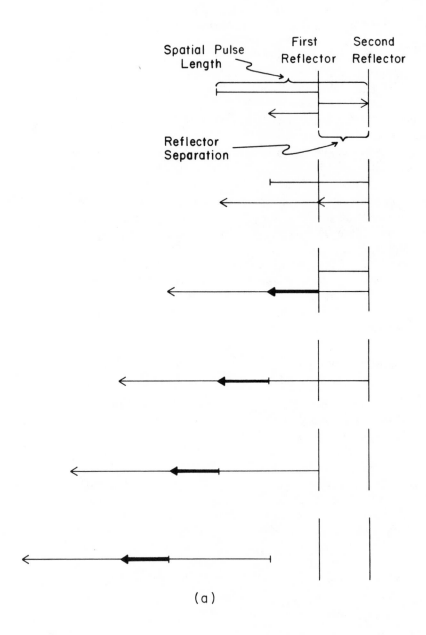

(a)

66

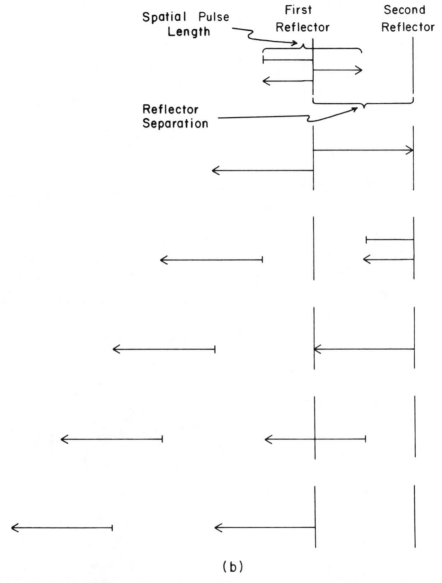

Figure 4.13. Axial resolution. (a) The separation of the reflectors is less than half the spatial pulse length, so that reflection overlap occurs. Separate reflections are not produced. The reflectors are not resolved. (b) The separation of the reflectors is greater than half the spatial pulse length, so that reflection overlap does not occur. Separate reflections are produced and the reflectors are resolved. Action proceeds in time from top to bottom in each part of the figure.

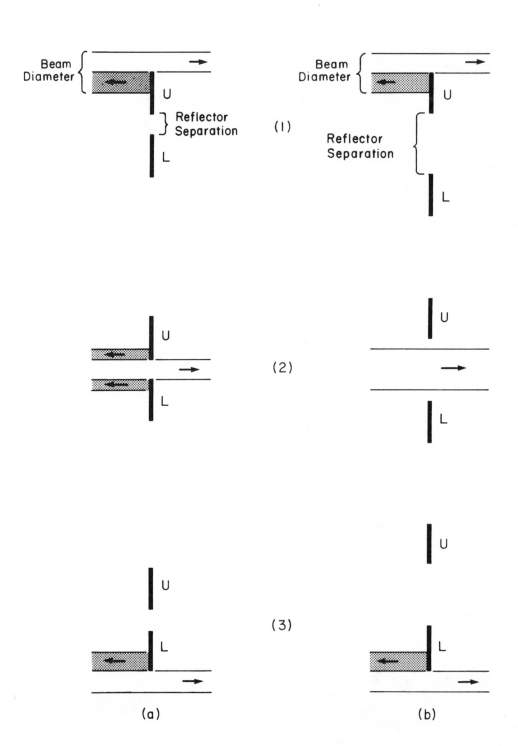

frequency. Recall that increasing the frequency also improves axial resolution, but at the expense of decreasing the half-intensity depth. A smaller transducer improves lateral resolution near the transducer, but makes it worse farther out (e.g., at 10 cm from the transducer in Figure 4.10). The primary means for reducing beam diameter and improving lateral resolution is focusing (Figure 4.11).

Diagnostic ultrasound transducers normally have better axial resolution than lateral resolution, although the two may be comparable in the focal region of highly focused beams. Imaging *system* resolution is normally not quite as good as transducer (acoustic) resolution discussed in this section. The resolution of the imaging system (ability to display detail) will be no better than the acoustic resolution. It may be slightly worse, because electronics and the display can degrade resolution.

Exercises

4.4.1. Axial resolution is the minimum reflector separation required along the direction of _____ _____ so that separate _____ are produced.

4.4.2. Axial resolution depends directly on _____ _____ _____ .

4.4.3. The smaller the axial resolution is, the better it is. True or false?

4.4.4. If there are three cycles of wavelength 1 mm in a pulse, the axial resolution is _____ mm.

4.4.5. For pulses traveling through soft tissue where frequency is 3 MHz and there are 4 cycles per pulse, the axial resolution is _____ mm.

Figure 4.14. Lateral resolution. (a) Reflector separation (perpendicular to beam direction) is less than beam diameter. (b) Reflector separation is greater than beam diameter. (1) Sound travels from left to right and encounters the upper reflector (U), with part of the beam (shaded) being reflected back toward the source and the remainder continuing past the reflector. (2) The beam has been scanned down so that (a) it is partially reflected by both upper and lower (L) reflectors or so that (b) no reflection occurs, the beam completely passing between the reflectors. (3) The beam has been scanned down further so that part of it is reflected by the lower reflector, the remainder continuing past the reflector. (a) The scanning sequence (1)-(2)-(3) results in continual reflection from one or both of the reflectors. Separate reflections are not produced, and the reflectors are not resolved. (b) The scanning sequence (1)-(2)-(3) results in reflection from the upper reflector, then no reflection, then reflection from the lower reflector. Separate reflections are produced, and the reflectors are resolved.

4.4.6. If there are three cycles per pulse, the axial resolution in soft tissue at the extremes of the useful frequency range for diagnostic ultrasound are _____ and _____ mm.

4.4.7. Doubling the frequency causes axial resolution to be _____ .

4.4.8. Doubling the number of cycles per pulse causes axial resolution to be _____ .

4.4.9. When studying an obese subject, a higher frequency will likely be required. True or false?

4.4.10. If better resolution is desired, a lower frequency will help. True or false?

4.4.11. If frequencies less than _____ MHz are used, axial resolution is not sufficient.

4.4.12. If frequencies higher than _____ MHz are used, half-intensity depth is not sufficient.

4.4.13. Increasing the frequency improves resolution because _____ is reduced, thus reducing _____ _____ _____ .

4.4.14. Increasing the frequency decreases the half-intensity depth because _____ is increased.

4.4.15. Lateral resolution is the minimum _____ between two reflectors such that when a beam is scanned across them, two separate _____ are produced.

4.4.16. Lateral resolution is equal to _____ _____ .

4.4.17. Lateral resolution is also called (more than one correct answer)
a. axial resolution
b. longitudinal resolution
c. angular resolution
d. azimuthal resolution
e. range resolution
f. transverse resolution
g. depth resolution

4.4.18. For a transducer of given diameter, increasing the frequency improves lateral resolution. True or false?

4.4.19. Lateral resolution varies with distance from the transducer. True or false?

4.4.20. For a given frequency, a smaller transducer always gives improved lateral resolution. True or false?

4.4.21. Lateral resolution is determined by (more than one correct
answer)
a. damping
b. frequency
c. transducer diameter
d. number of cycles in the pulse
e. distance from transducer
f. focusing

Transducers convert energy from one form to another. Ultrasound **4.5**
transducers convert electric energy to ultrasound energy and vice versa. **Review**
They operate on the piezoelectricity principle. Transducers may be
operated in continuous mode or pulsed mode. Axial resolution is equal
to one half the spatial pulse length. Pulsed transducers have damping
material to shorten the spatial pulse length. Disc transducers produce
sound in the form of beams with near and far zones. Lateral resolution
is equal to beam diameter. Beam diameter may be reduced by focusing.

Exercises

4.5.1. Match the following transducer assembly parts with their
functions:
a. cable: _____   1. reduces reflection at
b. damping material: _____   transducer surface
c. piezoelectric element: 2. converts voltage pulses
    _____   to sound pulses
d. matching layer: _____   3. reduces pulse duration
                                     4. conducts voltage pulses

4.5.2. Which of the following improve sound transmission from
the transducer element into the tissue? (More than one
correct answer.)
a. matching layer
b. Doppler effect
c. damping material
d. coupling medium
e. refraction

4.5.3. A transducer has a thickness of 0.4 mm, a diameter of 13
mm, and an element material propagation speed of 4 mm/
μs. Calculate the following:
a. operating frequency:
_____ MHz

    b. wavelength in soft tissue:

        _____ mm

    c. near-zone length in soft tissue:

        _____ mm

    d. lateral resolution at 14 cm:

        _____ mm

    e. lateral resolution at 28 cm:

        _____ mm

4.5.4. Lateral resolution is improved by
a. damping
b. pulsing
c. focusing
d. reflecting
e. absorbing

4.5.5. For an unfocused transducer, the best lateral resolution (minimum beam diameter) is _____ times the transducer diameter. This value of lateral resolution is found at a distance from the transducer face equal to the _____ length.

4.5.6. For a focused transducer, the best lateral resolution (minimum beam diameter) is found in the _____ region.

4.5.7. An unfocused 3.5-MHz 13-mm-diameter transducer will give a minimum beam diameter (best lateral resolution) of _____ mm.

4.5.8. An unfocused 3.5-MHz 13-mm-diameter transducer produces pulses of 3 cycles. The axial resolution in soft tissue is _____ mm.

4.5.9. In Problems 4.6.7 and 4.6.8, axial resolution is better than lateral resolution. True or false?

4.5.10. Axial resolution is often not as good as lateral resolution in diagnostic ultrasound. True or false?

4.5.11. The two resolutions may be comparable in the _____ region of a highly focused beam.

4.5.12. Beam diameter may be reduced in the near zone by focusing. True or false?

4.5.13. Beam diameter may be reduced in the far zone by focusing. True or false?

4.5.14. Match each transducer characteristic with the sound beam characteristic it determines (answers may be used more than once):

a. element thickness: _____,
    _____ and _____
b. element diameter: _____

1. axial resolution
2. lateral resolution
3. operating frequency

    c. element shape (flat or
       curved): _____
    d. damping: _____

4.5.15. The axial resolution of a transducer can be improved most by
    a. increasing the damping
    b. increasing the diameter
    c. decreasing the damping
    d. decreasing the frequency
    e. decreasing the diameter
    f. attaching a Dopple

4.5.16. The principle on which ultrasound transducers operate is the
    a. Doppler effect
    b. acousto-optic effect
    c. acoustoelectric effect
    d. cause and effect
    e. piezoelectric effect

4.5.17. Which of the following is *not* decreased by damping?
    a. refraction
    b. pulse duration
    c. spatial pulse length
    d. efficiency
    e. sensitivity

4.5.18. Which three things determine beam diameter for a disc transducer?
    a. pulse duration
    b. frequency
    c. disc diameter
    d. distance from disc face
    e. efficiency

4.5.19. A two-cycle pulse of 5-MHz ultrasound produces separate reflections from reflectors in soft tissue separated by 1 mm. True or false?

4.5.20. The lower and upper limits of the frequency range useful in diagnostic ultrasound are determined by _____ and _____ _____ _____ requirements, respectively.

4.5.21. The range of frequencies useful for diagnostic ultrasound is _____ to _____ MHz.

4.5.22. Since diagnostic ultrasound pulses are usually two or three cycles long, axial resolution is usually equal to _____ or _____ wavelengths.

Chapter 5

Static Imaging Instruments

5.1
Introduction

In the preceding chapters the process by which ultrasound is generated and how it interacts with tissues were described. The instruments that detect and present the information resulting from this interaction will now be considered. The pulse-echo method (Figure 5.1) uses received echoes. This method consists of ultrasound generation, propagation, and reflection in tissues and reception of returning reflections. Most diagnostic ultrasound systems in use today are the reflection (pulse-echo) type. These instruments detect three things: the strength, direction, and arrival time of reflections that occur in the tissues. This chapter describes what the instruments do with these quantities.

Imaging systems produce visual displays from the electric voltages received from the transducer. A diagram of the components of a pulse-echo imaging system is given in Figure 5.2. Several parameters that describe ultrasound were given in Chapters 2, 3, and 4. They are determined in this system as shown in Table 5.1.

Exercises

5.1.1. The five primary components of a diagnostic ultrasound imaging system are the _____ ,
_____ , _____ ,
_____ , and _____ .

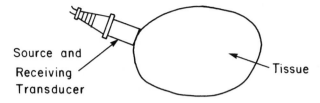

Figure 5.1. Diagnostic ultrasound pulse-echo information collection method. This method responds to reflection, attenuation, and propagation speed encountered in the tissue.

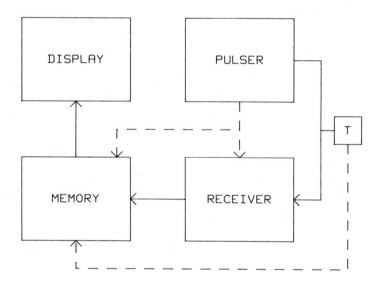

Figure 5.2. The components of a pulse-echo imaging system. The pulser produces electric pulses (Figure 5.3) that drive the transducer (T). It also produces pulses that tell the receiver and memory when the transducer has been driven. The transducer (acting as a source) produces an ultrasound pulse (Figure 5.3) for each electric pulse applied. For each reflection received from the tissues, an electric voltage is produced by the transducer (acting as a receiving transducer). These voltages go to the receiver, where they are processed to a form suitable for driving the memory. Information on transducer position (location) and orientation (which way it is pointing) is delivered (dash line) by electric voltages to the memory. Electric information from memory drives the display, which produces a visual image of the cross-sectional anatomy interrogated by the system.

75

Table 5.1
Determination of Ultrasound Parameters*

Ultrasound Parameter	Determined by
Frequency	transducer
Period	transducer
Wavelength	transducer, tissue
Propagation speed	tissue
Pulse repetition frequency	pulser
Pulse repetition period	pulser
Pulse duration	transducer
Duty factor	pulser, transducer
Spatial pulse length	transducer, tissue
Axial resolution	transducer, tissue
Amplitude	pulser, transducer
Intensity	pulser, transducer
Attenuation	transducer, tissue
Half-intensity depth	transducer, tissue
Beam diameter	transducer, tissue
Lateral resolution	transducer, tissue

*The ultrasound parameters described in Chapters 2, 3, and 4 are determined by imaging system components described in Chapters 4 and 5 (Figure 5.2). Overall imaging system axial and lateral resolutions are also determined by the receiver, memory, and display.

5.1.2. Match each component with its function:

a. pulser: _____
b. transducer: _____
c. receiver: _____
d. memory: _____
e. display: _____

1. produces ultrasound pulses
2. processes voltages received from the transducer
3. receives electric information from the memory
4. produces electric pulses that drive the transducer
5. provides electric information to the display

5.1.3. Match these ultrasound parameters produced by an instrument with the components that determine them (answers may be used more than once):

a. frequency: _____
b. period: _____
c. wavelength: _____ , _____

1. pulser
2. transducer
3. tissue

d. propagation speed _____

e. pulse repetition frequency: _____

f. pulse repetition period: _____

g. pulse duration: _____

h. duty factor: _____ , _____

i. spatial pulse length: _____ , _____

j. axial resolution: _____ , _____

k. amplitude: _____ , _____

l. intensity: _____ , _____

m. attenuation: _____ , _____

n. half-intensity depth: _____ , _____

o. beam diameter: _____ , _____

p. lateral resolution: _____ , _____

5.2 Pulser

The pulser is where the action originates. It produces electric voltage pulses (Figure 5.3) that (1) drive the transducer, which produces ultrasound pulses, and (2) tells the receiver and memory when the ultrasound pulses are produced. The pulse repetition frequency of the pulser is the number of electrical pulses produced per second. It is typically 1000 Hz or 1 kHz. The ultrasound pulse repetition frequency is equal to the voltage pulse repetition frequency, since one ultrasound pulse is produced for each voltage pulse (Figure 5.3). Similarly, the ultrasound pulse repetition period is equal to the voltage pulse repetition period. The voltage pulse duration is much less than the period of the cycles in the ultrasound pulses. To receive information for display at a rapid rate, it is necessary to use a high repetition frequency. Repetition frequency, however, must be limited in order to provide an unambiguous display of returning reflections. This is described in Chapter 8. The timing sequence that is initiated by the pulser is shown in Figure 5.4.

The greater the pulse amplitude produced by the pulser, the greater will be the amplitude and intensity of the ultrasound pulses produced by the transducer. Ultrasound pulse amplitude and intensity depend also on the transducer efficiency. Electric pulse amplitudes are generally a few tens or hundreds of volts.

Table 5.2 gives typical ranges for acoustic outputs of diagnostic instruments.

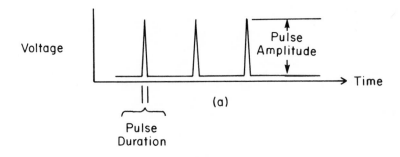

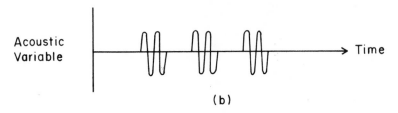

Figure 5.3. An ultrasound pulse (b) is produced by the transducer for every voltage pulse (a) applied.

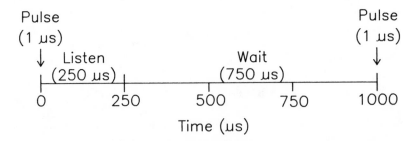

Figure 5.4. Timing sequence for pulse-echo ultrasound imaging. The sequence is initiated by the production of a 1-μs pulse of ultrasound when the pulser sends a voltage pulse to the transducer. This is followed by a period of up to 250 μs during which echoes are received from the tissue by the transducer. The length of this time is determined by the maximum depth from which the echoes return. For example, for 2 MHz, echoes can return from as deep as 20 cm. The round-trip travel time to this depth is 260 μs. This listening period is followed by a waiting period until the next pulse is produced. In this illustration, the waiting period is 750 μs. Here, the pulse repetition period is 1000 μs (pulse repetition frequency 1 kHz). If the pulse repetition frequency were greater, the pulse repetition period would be less, resulting in a shorter waiting period.

Table 5.2 79

Ranges for Acoustic Output Parameters of Diagnostic
Ultrasound Imaging Instruments[11–13]

Parameter	Range
SATA intensity	0.06–60 mW/cm^2
SPTA intensity	0.01–200 mW/cm^2
SPTP intensity	0.5–280 W/cm^2
Beam uniformity ratio	
Unfocused	2–3
Focused	5–200
Duty factor	0.001–0.003
Cycles per pulse	2–6
Pulse repetition frequency	0.5–3 kHz

Exercises

5.2.1. The ultrasound pulse repetition frequency is equal to the
voltage _____repetition frequency of the
pulser.

5.2.2. Increased pulse amplitude produced by the pulser increases
the _____ and _____ of
ultrasound pulses produced by the transducer.

5.2.3. Match these acoustic parameters produced by diagnostic
instruments with their typical values:
a. SATA intensity: _____   1. 50
b. SPTP intensity: _____   2. 0.001
c. beam uniformity ratio: _____   3. 1 mW/cm^2
d. duty factor: _____   4. 3
e. cycles per pulse: _____   5. 1 W/cm^2

Voltages produced in the transducer by returning reflections are sent **5.3**
to the receiver for processing. The receiver performs the following **Receiver**
functions:

1. **amplification**
2. **compensation**
3. **demodulation**
4. **compression**
5. **rejection**

Amplification is increasing the small voltages received from the transducer to larger ones suitable for processing and storage (Figure 5.5). **Gain** is the ratio of output to input of electric power. The power ratio is equal to the square of the voltage ratio (across the same resistance); power ratio may be expressed in decibels (Appendix C). For example, if the input voltage amplitude to an **amplifier** is 2 mV and the ouput voltage amplitude is 200 mV, the voltage ratio is 200/2 or 100. The power ratio is $(100)^2$ or 10,000. From Table C.2 the power ratio or gain is found to be 40 dB. Receiver amplifiers usually have 60–100 dB of gain. Voltages applied to these amplifiers range from tens of microvolts to tens of millivolts.

In some systems that have long cables connecting the transducer to the internal electronics of the instrument, part of the amplification is performed by a **preamplifier** located close to the transducer. Preamplification increases the voltages from the transducer relative to the electric noise picked up along the cable to the instrument.

Compensation (also called gain compensation, swept gain, time gain compensation, or depth gain compensation) equalizes differences in received reflection amplitudes because of reflector depth. Reflectors with equal reflection coefficients (Section 3.2) will not result in equal amplitude reflections arriving at the transducer (Figure 5.6) if their travel distances are different (distances from the transducer to the reflectors are different). This is because attenuation depends on path length (Section 2.5). It is desirable to display reflections from reflectors of equal reflection coefficients, sizes, and shapes in a similar way. Since these reflections may not arrive with the same amplitude, because of different path lengths, their amplitudes must be adjusted to compensate for path length differences. Larger path lengths result in later arrival times. Therefore, if voltages from reflections arriving later are amplified more than earlier ones, attenuation compensation is accomplished. This is what compensation does (Figure 5.7).

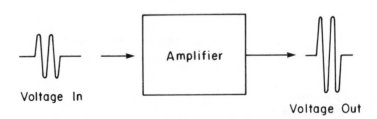

Voltage In

Amplifier

Voltage Out

Figure 5.5. Amplification increases voltage amplitude and electrical power.

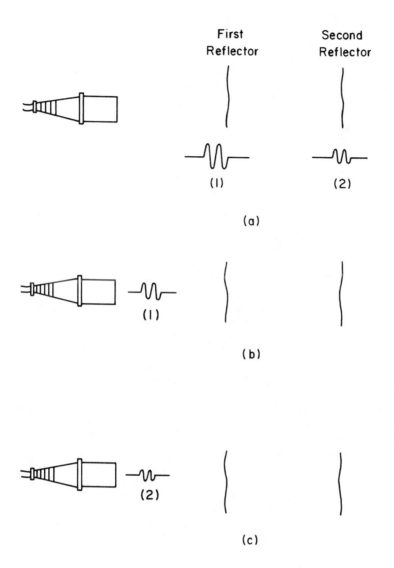

Figure 5.6. Two reflectors with equal reflection coefficients but different distances from the transducer. (a) The reflected pulse at the second reflector is weaker because the incident pulse has to travel farther to get to the second reflector, thus experiencing more attenuation. (b) The reflection from the first reflector arrives at the transducer. It is weaker than it was in (a) because of attenuation on the return trip. (c) The reflection from the second reflector arrives at the transducer later and weaker than the first one did. This is because of the longer path to the second reflector.

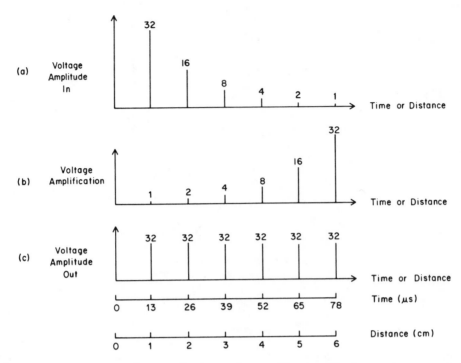

Figure 5.7. Compensation of attenuation by varying amplification. The time scale represents the arrival time of reflections. The distance scale represents the distance from the transducer to the reflectors. (a) Arriving reflections produce different voltage amplitudes because of attenuation. All reflections are assumed here to have come from reflectors with equal reflection coefficients. Each reflection arrives 13 μs after the previous one, and thus for soft tissue each reflector is 1 cm farther from the transducer (Problem 3.5.6). Each reflection produces a voltage amplitude one-half that of the previous one in this example. (b) Amplification must compensate for this by doubling as each 13 μs of time passes during the arrival of the reflections. Each arriving voltage amplitude (a) times the gain or amplification (b) existing at the time the voltage arrives at the amplifier equals the voltage amplitude out of the amplifier (c). Following this process, all the voltages are equalized. This is the case where all reflections result from equal reflection coefficients. If reflection coefficients of the various reflectors are different, the resulting voltage amplitudes, even after compensation, will be different. These differences should not be normalized or information would be lost.

Demodulation (sometimes called detection or envelope detection) is the process of converting the voltages delivered to the receiver from one form to another (Figure 5.8). This is done by rectification and smoothing (filtering) (Figure 5.9).

Compression is the process of decreasing the differences between the smallest and largest amplitudes (Figure 5.10). This is accomplished by logarithmic amplifiers that amplify weak inputs more than strong

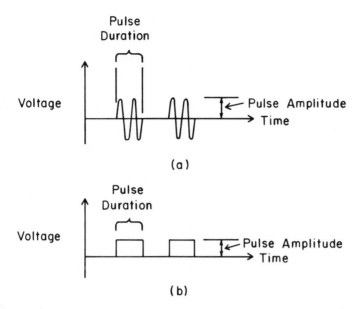

Figure 5.8. Demodulation is the conversion of pulses (a) to another form (b). Pulse amplitudes in (a) and (b) are proportional to each other. Ideally, pulse durations in (a) and (b) are equal to each other. In practice, there is some lengthening of the pulse duration during demodulation.

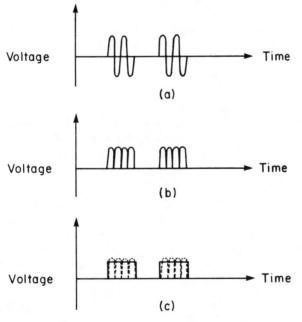

Figure 5.9. Rectification (b) and smoothing (filtering) (c) of pulses (a) results in demodulation (see Figure 5.8).

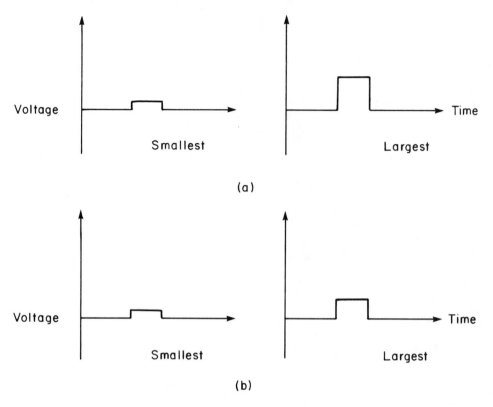

Figure 5.10. Compression decreases the difference between the smallest and the largest voltages passing through the system. In this illustration, (a) before compression the ratio of the largest to smallest amplitudes is five. (b) After compression the ratio is three.

ones. The ratio of the largest power to the smallest power that the system can handle is called the **dynamic range**. It is expressed in decibels. For example, if an amplifier is insensitive to voltage amplitudes less than 0.01 mV and cannot properly handle voltage amplitudes greater than 1000 mV, the ratio of voltages is 1000/0.01 or 100,000. The power ratio is equal to the square of the voltage ratio: $(100,000)^2$ or 10,000,000,000. According to Table C.2, the dynamic range of the amplifier is 100 dB. Although amplifiers have such a dynamic range, demodulators and displays do not. Their dynamic ranges are approximately 40 and 20 dB, respectively. The largest power can be only 100 times the smallest for the display. Thus, the largest voltage amplitude can only be 10 times the smallest. The dynamic range remaining after compensation is typically 40 dB. A compressor would have to compress the voltage ratio (100) corresponding to 40 dB to a voltage ratio of 10 (acceptable for the display).

Rejection (sometimes called suppression or threshold) eliminates the smaller-amplitude voltage pulses produced by weaker reflections or electronic noise (Figure 5.11). The weaker reflections often come from multiple scattering from within the tissue, thus constituting "acoustic noise." It is desirable to eliminate noise, electronic or acoustic, from the image, since it contributes no useful information and interferes with the observation of the useful information that *is* presented.

Figure 5.12 summarizes the five receiver functions discussed. The amplification (gain), compensation, and rejection functions are normally operator-adjustable; demodulation and compression are not.

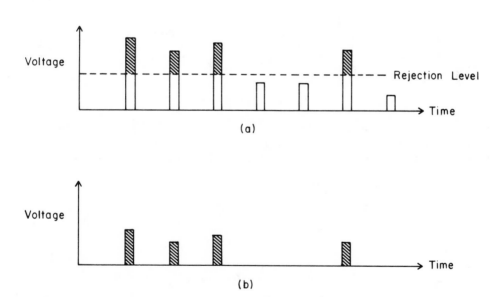

Figure 5.11. Rejection eliminates voltage pulses with amplitudes below the rejection level. (a) Before rejection. (b) After rejection.

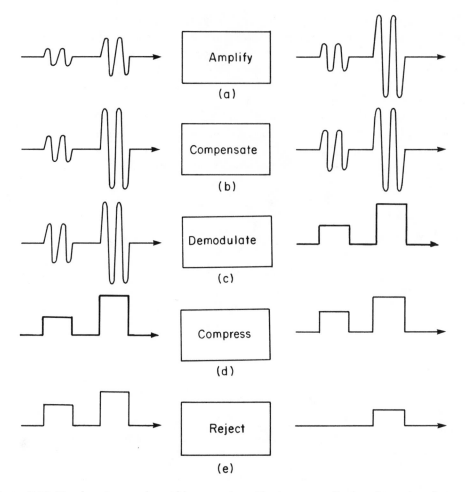

Figure 5.12. Five functions performed by a receiver. The larger-amplitude pulse arrives first. (a) Both pulses are amplified, doubling their amplitudes in this example. (b) The latter (weaker) pulse is amplified more. (c) The pulses are converted to another form. (d) The difference between the pulse amplitudes is reduced. (e) The weaker pulse is rejected because it is not above the rejection level.

Exercises

5.3.1. Five functions performed by the receiver are

_____ , _____ ,

_____ , _____ , and

_____ .

5.3.2. Match the following functions with what they accomplish:
    a. amplification: _____   1. converts pulses from one
    b. compensation: _____   form to another
    c. demodulation: _____   2. increases all amplitudes
    d. compression: _____   3. decreases dynamic range
    e. rejection: _____   4. eliminates some pulses
                                 5. corrects for tissue
                                    attenuation

5.3.3. Input voltage to an amplifier is 1 mV and output voltage is 10 mV. The voltage amplification ratio is _____ . The power ratio is _____ . The gain is _____ dB.

5.3.4. A receiver with a gain of 60 dB has 1 μW of power applied to the input. The output power is _____watt(s).

5.3.5. A receiver with a gain of 60 dB has 10 μV of voltage applied to the input. The output voltage is _____ mV.

5.3.6. Compensation is also called (more than one correct answer)
    a. swept beam
    b. swept gain
    c. refraction
    d. diffraction
    e. time gain compensation

5.3.7. Compensation takes into account reflector _____ or _____ .

5.3.8. Compensation amplifies pulses differently, according to their arrival _____ .

5.3.9. Compression decreases the _____ range to a range that the _____ can handle.

5.3.10. If a display has a dynamic range of 20 dB and the smallest voltage it can handle is 200 mV, the largest voltage it can handle is _____V.

5.3.11. Demodulation converts voltage _____ from one form to another.

5.3.12. Rejection eliminates higher-amplitude pulses. True or false?

5.3.13. Another name for rejection is
    a. threshold
    b. depth gain compensation
    c. swept gain
    d. compression
    e. demodulation

5.4
Memory

For **static imaging** (single **frame** imaging*), the echo information acquired as the transducer is passed over the patient must be stored.

Two types of image memories are used in diagnostic ultrasound instruments—**analog** and **digital.** These memories are commonly called **scan converters** because they provide a means for displaying, using a television scan format (Section 5.5), information acquired by a linear, sector, or manual transducer scanning technique (Section 5.5 and Chapter 6). The image plane is divided into squares called **pixels** (picture elements), commonly 1000 × 1000 or 2000 × 2000 (analog), 512 × 512 (square format digital), or 512 × 640 (rectangular format digital) squares on a side. In each of these spaces an electric charge (analog) or a number (digital) is stored that corresponds to the echo intensity received from the point within the body corresponding to that storage position.

The analog scan converter consists of a square matrix of electrical insulators, 1000 or 2000 on each side (1,000,000 or 4,000,000 total). An electron beam is directed toward this matrix [Figure 5.13 (a)] and is swept across it in a direction corresponding to the direction in which the ultrasound passes through the anatomy [Figure 5.13 (b)]. The current in the electron beam is increased and decreased corresponding to the increasing and decreasing intensity of the series of echoes that comes back to the transducer as the transmitted ultrasound pulse travels through the tissue. This results in various electric charge strengths being stored in the individual storage elements of the analog scan converter. After a single ultrasound pulse has traveled through the tissue in a given path, the information corresponding to the returned echoes is stored along a corresponding path in the scan converter in the form of various electric charge values in the insulator elements along that path [Figure 5.13 (b)].

A digital scan converter is a computer memory that stores numbers. As in the analog scan converter, a matrix of digital memory elements is used to store echo information. Either a square matrix, 512 on a side (262,144 total), or a rectangular matrix, 512 × 640 (327,680 total), is used. In each of these elements a number is stored corresponding to the echo intensity received from the point within the body corresponding to that storage position (Figure 5.14). If the digital memory were made up of a single matrix checkerboard, each pixel could only store one of two numbers, a zero or a one. This is because such memories are binary in nature and can only operate in two conditions, on or off, corresponding to one or zero. This would allow **bistable** or black and white imaging. In order to image **gray scale** (several shades of gray or brightness in addition to black and white), it is necessary to have more than one checkerboard. In a four-**bit** (binary digit) memory

*Dynamic imaging (rapid frame sequence imaging) is described in Chapter 6.

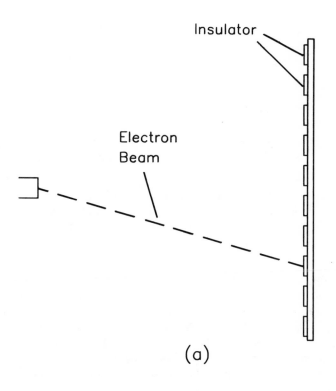

Insulator

Electron
Beam

(a)

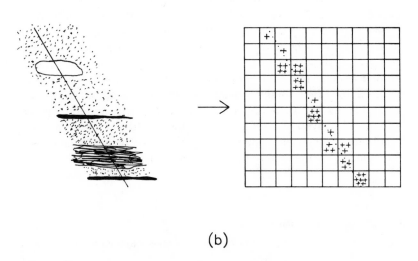

(b)

Figure 5.13. Analog scan converter. (a) (Side view.) A square matrix of insulators is scanned by an electron beam as the patient is scanned by the ultrasound beam. (b) (Anatomy cross-section scanned and front view of scan converter.) Electric charge is stored on the insulators in proportion to the intensity of the echoes received from corresponding anatomic locations.

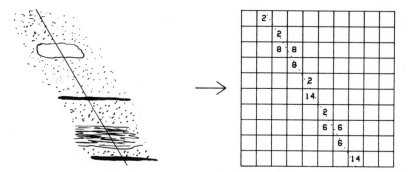

Figure 5.14. Anatomy cross-section scanned and front view of digital scan converter. Numbers are stored in the memory elements according to the intensity of the echoes received from corresponding anatomic locations.

there are four checkerboards back to back so that each pixel has four bits associated with it. In the binary numbering system (Appendix C) this allows numbers from 0 to 15 (16-shade system) to be stored. Other examples are given in Table 5.3. A 10 × 10, four-bit (per pixel) memory is shown in Figure 5.15. The total number of memory elements in various digital memories is given in Table 5.4.

The procedure for storing the information required for display of the two-dimensional cross-sectional image for either analog or digital scan converters is as follows: the transducer is scanned over the surface of the patient in such a way that the ultrasound beam "cuts" through the tissue in cross section. Echoes received from all points on this cross section are converted to electrical charges or numbers, which are stored at corresponding places in the analog or digital memory. All the information necessary for displaying this cross-sectional image is then stored in memory. The information can then be taken out of memory and applied to a two-dimensional display (cathode ray tube; Section 5.5) and displayed in such a way that the electrical charge values or numbers coming out of memory are displayed with corresponding brightnesses on the face of the tube (Figure 5.16.)

Table 5.3
Characteristics of Digital Memories

Number of Bits	Lowest Number Stored	Highest Number Stored	Shades
4	0	15	16
5	0	31	32
6	0	63	64
7	0	127	128
8	0	255	256

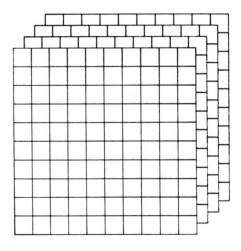

Figure 5.15. A 10 × 10 pixel, four-bit deep (4 bits per pixel) digital memory.

Table 5.4
Bits (Binary Digits or Memory Elements) in Digital Memories

Dimensions	Pixels	Bits Deep	Total Bits
512 × 512	262,144	4	1,050,000
512 × 512	262,144	5	1,310,000
512 × 512	262,144	6	1,570,000
512 × 512	264,144	7	1,840,000
512 × 640	327,680	4	1,310,000
512 × 640	327,680	5	1,640,000
512 × 640	327,680	6	1,970,000
512 × 640	327,680	7	2,290,000

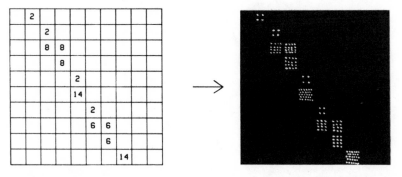

Figure 5.16. For display of scanned anatomy, numbers are read out of pixel locations in digital memory and applied to the display in such a way that brightness corresponds to stored number.

Analog is derived from the Greek for "proportionate" and digital from Latin for "finger" or "toe." Analog scan converters are continuous in nature, that is, they can store any value of charge in each pixel from the minimum to the maximum capability of the device. Digital scan converters are discrete, that is they can only store whole numbers in each pixel location from zero to a maximum that is determined by the number of bits per pixel (Table 5.3).

For a 1000 × 1000 memory matrix in which the represented anatomic depth is 20 cm, each pixel represents anatomic dimensions of 0.2 mm. For a 512 × 512 matrix the result is 0.4 mm. This represents the spatial resolution of the memory matrix. If the maximum depth represented in memory is 10 cm, then the memory spatial resolutions are 0.1 and 0.2 mm, respectively. The 512 × 640 rectangular matrix is sometimes used because it is more representive of the oval shape of the normal abdomen cross section in which the anterior-posterior dimension is about 80 percent of the lateral dimension.

Preprocessing, in digital systems, is the assignment of specific numbers to echo intensities as they are stored in memory (Figure 5.17). Postprocessing is the assignment of specific display brightnesses to

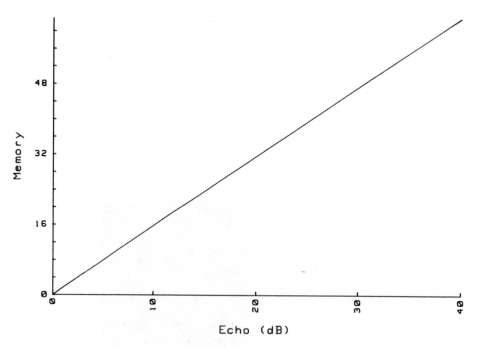

Figure 5.17. Digital preprocessing is the assignment of numbers (to be stored in memory) to echo intensities. Here echo intensity is expressed in decibels (relative to the weakest echo, which is represented as 0 dB. Forty decibels is the strongest echo—10,000 times the intensity of the weakest).

numbers coming out of memory (Figure 5.18). For most digital systems, the preprocessing scheme is a linear one (Figure 5.17) and cannot be controlled by the operator. For a linear preprocessing assignment, the echo dynamic range is equally divided throughout the gray levels of the system. Table 5.5 gives, for four to seven bit systems, the number of decibels per shade (assuming a 40-dB echo dynamic range after attenuation compensation) and the average intensity difference between two echoes in order for them to be assigned to different shades (number in memory) in the system. This is known as **gray-scale resolution**. For a four-bit system, an echo must have nearly twice the intensity of another one for them to get assigned different shades. For a seven-bit system, only a 7-percent difference is required. On many instruments, one of several preprogrammed postprocessing schemes is selectable by the operator. On others, the postprocessing curve may be designed as desired by the operator using panel controls. A linear assignment (Figure 5.18) equally divides the display brightness range among the stored gray levels of the system. Other schemes (Figure 5.19) may be used that allow assignment of more of the brightness range to certain portions of the stored-number range capability of the system. Figure

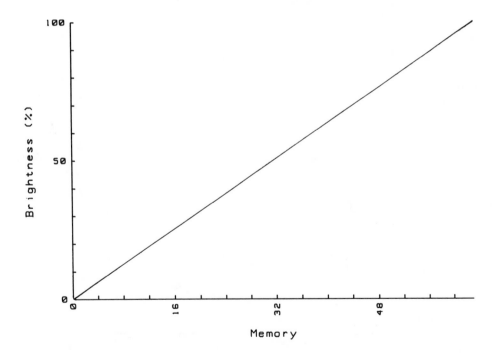

Figure 5.18. Digital postprocessing is the assignment of specific display brightnesses to numbers coming out of specific pixel locations in memory.

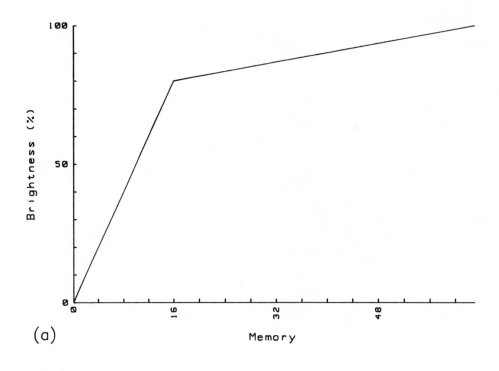

(a)

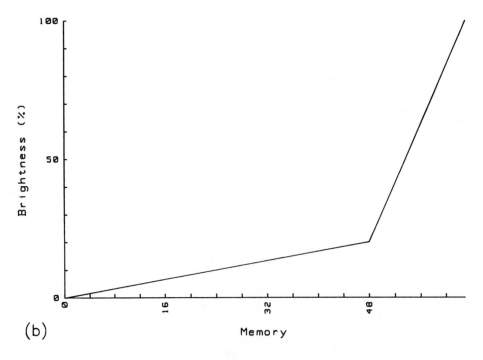

(b)

94

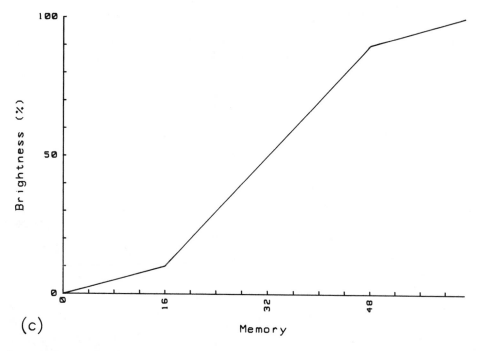

(c)

Figure 5.19. Postprocessing assignment schemes. A large brightness range is reserved for (a) weak, (b) strong, and (c) intermediate echoes.

5.19 (a) represents one of the most useful schemes, which assigns more gray scale range to the weaker echoes that result from scattering and are therefore angle-independent (Section 3.4).

Most digital instruments digitize the electrical voltages coming out of the receiver. However, some digitize earlier in the process, allowing some receiver functions to be carried out digitally, e.g., demodulation.

Table 5.5
Gray-Scale Resolution of Digital Memories*

Bits per Pixel	Decibels per Shade	Intensity Difference (%)[†]
4	2.5	78
5	1.2	32
6	0.6	15
7	0.3	7

*assuming a 40-dB echo dynamic range.
[†] The average difference required between two echoes in order for them to be assigned to different shades.

95

5.4.1. For the digital memory shown in Figure 5.20, match pixel locations with numbers stored:

a. lower right: _____   1. 13
b. middle right: _____   2. 10
c. upper right: _____   3. 9
d. upper middle: _____   4. 14
e. upper left: _____   5. 6

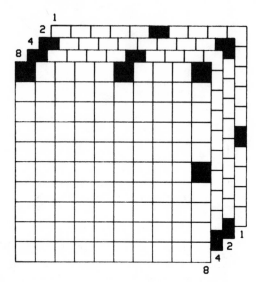

Figure 5.20. Digital memory description for Problem 5.4.1. Blank indicates that the memory device is on.

5.4.2. The gray-scale resolution for a digital instrument that has an echo dynamic range of 43 dB and 32 shades is _____ dB per shade.
a. 1.3
b. 3.2
c. 4.3
d. 32
e. 43

5.4.3. The gray-scale resolution for a 6-bit digital instrument that has an echo dynamic range of 45 dB is _____ .
a. 0.3
b. 0.5
c. 0.7
d. 0.9
e. 6

5.4.4. Match the following:

a. analog: _____   1. picture element
b. digital: _____   2. assignment of stored numbers
c. preprocessing: _____   3. discrete
d. postprocessing: _____   4. binary digit
e. pixel: _____   5. continuous
f. bit: _____   6. assignment of displayed
                                                 brightnesses

5.4.5. Typical digital pixel matrix dimensions are _____ .

a. 640 × 128
b. 16 × 64
c. 100 × 100
d. 512 × 1540
e. 512 × 512

5.4.6. Match the number of shades with bits per pixel:

a. 16: _____   1. 1
                                   2. 2
b. 32: _____   3. 3
                                   4. 4
c. 64: _____   5. 5
                                   6. 6
d. 128: _____   7. 7
                                   8. 8
e. 256: _____   9. 9
                                 10. 10

5.4.7. _____ total memory elements are required for a 100 × 100 pixel, 5-bit digital memory.

a. 100
b. 10,000
c. 500
d. 50,000
e. 100,000

5.4.8. Analog scan converters store information in terms of _____ .

a. logarithms
b. electric magnetism
c. electric current
d. electric charge
e. numbers

5.4.9. Digital scan converters store _____ .

a. logarithms
b. electric magnetism
c. electric current
d. electric charge
e. numbers

5.4.10. _____ is commonly controllable by the operator.
  a. postprocessing
  b. gray-scale resolution
  c. bits per pixel
  d. digitization
  e. all of the above

**5.5
Display**

There are several ways in which the information delivered to the display may be presented. Those in common use are:

1. **A mode**
2. **B mode**
3. **M mode**
4. **B scan**

The display device used in each case is a **cathode-ray tube.** This tube generates a sharply focused beam of electrons that produces a bright spot on the phosphor-coated front face (screen) of the tube (Figure 5.21). This spot can be moved across or up and down the face by applying voltages to deflection plates (Figure 5.22) or electric currents to magnetic deflection coils. If the voltage or current is properly varied, the spot can be made to move across the face at a constant speed. At the completion of this motion (i.e., when a **scan line** is completed), the spot can be made to jump rapidly back to the starting point.

Amplitude-mode (A-mode) operation causes a vertical deflection of the spot each time a pulse is delivered from the receiver (i.e., each time a reflection is received by the transducer). The horizontal position

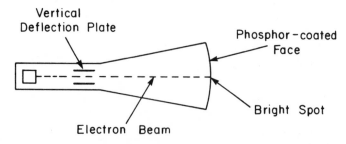

Figure 5.21. A cathode-ray tube (side view). The electron beam produces a bright spot where it strikes the phosphor-coated face of the tube. There is a set of horizontal deflection plates that is not shown.

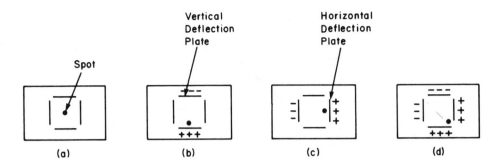

Figure 5.22. Spot deflection on the face of a cathode-ray tube (front view). (a) No voltage is applied to deflection plates; the spot is centered. (b) Voltage is applied to vertical deflection plates; the spot is deflected down. Increasing the voltage increases the deflection. If applied voltage were reversed, the spot would be deflected up. (c) Voltage is applied to horizontal deflection plates; the spot is deflected to the right. (d) Voltage is applied to both sets of plates; the spot is deflected down and to the right.

of the vertical deflection (Figure 5.23) is determined by pulse travel time (and thus by reflector distance). The vertical deflection amplitude is determined by the received reflection amplitude and by the amplification, compensation, compression, and rejection of the receiver. The A mode is commonly used in setting up M-mode presentations.

Brightness mode (B-mode) operation causes a brightening of the spot rather than a deflection each time a reflection is received (Figure 5.24). Back-and-forth motion of the reflector is seen as back-and-forth motion of the vertical deflection in the A mode or the bright spot in the B mode.

Motion mode (M-mode) operation is B mode operation in which the motion of the spots is recorded by a recording medium (strip chart recorder) that moves across the face of the display. This results in a recording of the reflector motion (Figure 5.24). The M mode is commonly used in heart studies.

B-scan (B-mode-scan) operation causes a brightening of the spot, as in the B and M modes. However, the scan lines are not horizontal, as they are in these modes. The starting point and direction of motion across the face are determined in the B mode by the position and orientation of the transducer (Figure 5.25). An image (B scan) of the object scanned may be built up on the face of the tube as the transducer is moved through many locations and orientations (Figure 5.26). Some means of storing echo information during this scanning must be provided. This was discussed in the previous section. The B scan is an image that is a cross section of the object through the scanning plane, as if the sound beam were cutting a section through the tissues (a tomogram).

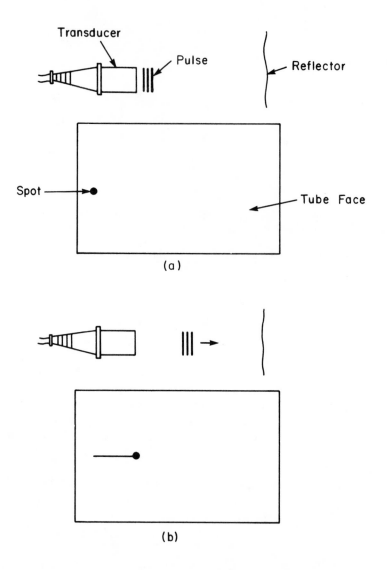

Figure 5.23. A-mode presentation of a reflection. (a) As the pulse leaves the transducer, the spot on the face of the cathode-ray tube begins to move to the right. (b) As the pulse moves toward the reflector, the spot continues to move to the right. (c) When the pulse is reflected, the spot has moved across the face an amount corresponding to half the transducer–reflector separation. (d) The spot continues to move to the right as the reflection moves toward the transducer. (e) When the reflection arrives at the transducer, an electric pulse is delivered to the receiver, which delivers an electric pulse to the display. This is applied to vertical deflection plates, causing the spot to deflect up at a horizontal position corresponding to the transducer–reflector separation. This process is repeated each time a pulse is delivered from the pulser to the transducer. A system with no memory is assumed in this description. Memory is not necessary in A-mode presentations.

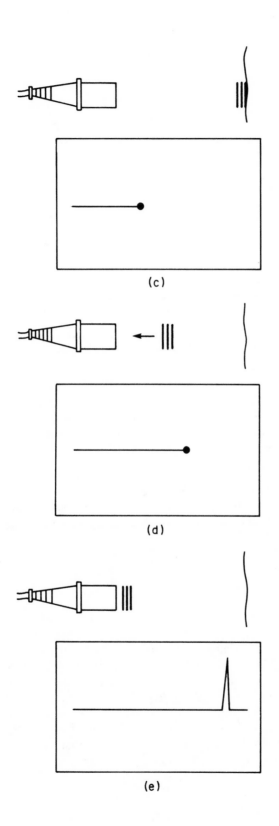

(c)

(d)

(e)

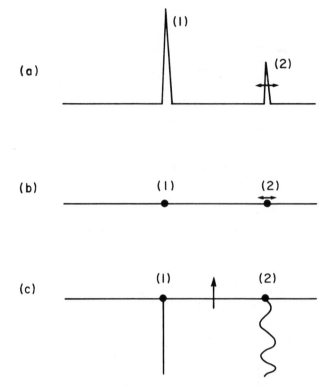

Figure 5.24. Three presentations of a reflection. Reflection 1 is produced at a stationary reflector. Reflection 2 is produced at a deeper reflector that is moving back and forth. (a) Vertical deflection 2 in the A mode moves left and right as the reflector moves closer to and farther from the transducer. (b) The bright spot 2 in the B mode moves left and right as the reflector moves closer to and farther from the transducer. (c) As the process is repeated and a recording medium is moved across the face of the display, the motion of reflector 2 is traced out in the M mode.

The transducer is attached to an articulated (Latin: jointed) scanning arm to confine the scanning motion and the beam path through the tissue to a plane. Information regarding transducer position and orientation during the scan must be sent to the memory or display. This information comes from devices at the joints of the scan arm sections (Figure 5.27). These devices are either potentiometers (variable **electrical resistors**) or optical encoders (devices that count light pulses with changing angle).

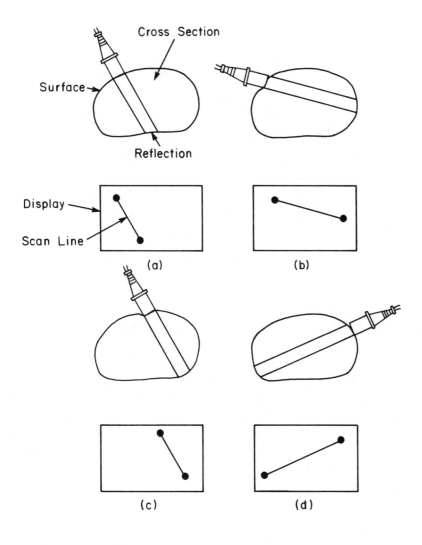

Figure 5.25. B-scan presentation of a reflection. (a) The transducer is shown in one location pointing in one direction. The reflection produces a bright spot on the display, as shown. (b) The transducer is in the same location as in (a), but it is pointing in another direction. The starting point for the scan line on the display is the same as in (a), but the line points in a different direction (the direction in which the transducer is pointing). (c) The transducer is in a location different from its locations in (a) and (b), but it is pointing in a direction parallel to that in (a). (d) The transducer is in a new location and is pointed in a different direction. By manually placing the transducer in many locations and orientations, a complete image (B scan) of the object is built up on the display (Figure 5.26). Memory is required to do this (Section 5.4).

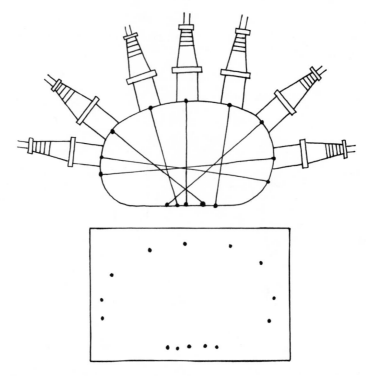

Figure 5.26. Building up a B-mode image (B scan) by moving the transducer through many locations and orientations.

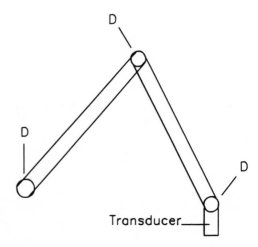

Figure 5.27. An articulated scanning arm for B-scan imaging. (D) Potentiometers or optical encoders send transducer location and orientation information to the memory or display.

For many years diagnostic ultrasound displays used cathode-ray storage tubes that could not display various brightnesses. The amplitude of the pulse delivered by the receiver had little effect on the brightness of the spot displayed. The bright spots either were there or were not there. This is referred to as **bistable display** (on or off). In common use now is **gray-scale display,** in which several values of brightness may be stored and displayed. These displays produce B-scan presentations in which brightness is determined by received reflection amplitude. Higher-amplitude reflections may be presented as brighter (white echo) spots or as darker (black echo) spots. In some instruments, either display method may be chosen.

The scan converter (Section 5.4) is a device that has made stored gray-scale displays possible. It stores the gray-scale image and allows it to be displayed on a television monitor. Gray-scale presentation of reflections preserves some of their dynamic range. Scan converters are capable of storing a greater dynamic range of brightness than the eye can handle. However, photography of displayed images usually limits the dynamic range to less than that of the eye.

M-mode display is usually recorded by a strip-chart recorder. B-scan displays are usually recorded by photography. Real-time displays (see Chapter 6) are recorded on videotape or disc.

For measurement purposes, most displays include range marker dots or calipers or both. Marker dots are presented as a series of dots in a line with given separation (e.g., 1 cm). Calipers are two pluses (or some other symbol) which can be placed anywhere on the display. The distance between them is calculated by the instrument and read out on the display.

Television monitors are commonly used as the display devices for static and dynamic ultrasound imaging instruments. A television monitor is a cathode-ray tube in which a particular electron beam scanning format is utilized. The electron beam current is continually changed as the beam is scanned to provide varying brightness of the spot, thus providing gray-scale imaging capability. The television scanning format consists of a left-to-right and top-to-bottom scanning pattern similar to the way in which this page of written text is read. The resulting display consists of 525 horizontal display scan lines that produce the static image or one frame of a dynamic image. This picture is rewritten (static imaging) repeatedly or updated (dynamic imaging) 30 times each second. This compares to motion picture film in which 24 frames per second are used.

Exercises

5.5.1 The common methods of image presentation are called
_____ mode, _____ mode, _____ mode, and _____
scan.

5.5.2 Match the following display modes with the appropriate statements (answers may be used more than once):

a. A mode: _____ , _____

b. B mode: _____ , _____

c. M mode: _____ , _____ , _____

d. B scan: _____ , _____ , _____ , _____

1. cross-sectional display
2. dot is deflected by return of a reflection
3. dot is brightened by return of a reflection
4. one axis of recording corresponds to time
5. scan lines move with transducer position and orientation
6. requires the transducer to be moved or scanned to develop the image
7. gives a one-dimensional display

5.5.3. The display device used in each mode is a _____ tube.

5.5.4. The spot on a cathode-ray tube may be moved by applying voltage to the _____ plates.

5.5.5. In the A mode, the horizontal position of the vertical deflection is determined by pulse travel _____ and thus by reflector _____ .

5.5.6. In the A mode, a vertical deflection nearer the left-hand side of the tube face results from a reflector that is nearer the transducer. True or false?

5.5.7. The _____ mode is used for studying the motion of a reflector.

5.5.8. To position a bright spot on the display in the B mode, the instrument uses the arrival _____ of the reflection and must assume a value for _____ _____ in tissue.

5.5.9. The B scan presents a cross section through the _____ plane.

5.5.10. A display that preserves some of the reflector dynamic range is called a _____ display.

5.5.11. The _____ _____ stores the gray-scale image and allows it to be displayed on a television monitor.

5.5.12. Television monitors produce _____ images per second.
a. 10
b. 15

    c. 30

    d. 60

    e. 100

5.5.13. How many horizontal lines are used to produce a picture on a television monitor?

    a. 60

    b. 100

    c. 256

    d. 525

    e. 1024

5.5.14. It takes _____ ms of time to produce a single picture on a television monitor using the television scan format.

5.5.15. It takes _____ μs of time to write one horizontal line of brightness information on a television monitor.

5.6 Review

Diagnostic ultrasound imaging systems are of the reflection (pulse-echo) type. These use the direction, strength, and arrival time of received reflections to generate a one-dimensional A-mode or M-mode display or to generate a two-dimensional gray-scale B-mode display. Imaging systems consist of a pulser, a transducer, a receiver, a memory, and a display. Receivers amplify, compensate, demodulate, compress, and reject. Compensation equalizes differences in received reflection amplitudes caused by reflector depth. The A mode uses a deflection display. The M and B modes use a brightness display. The M mode shows reflector motion in time. The B scan shows a cross section through the scanning plane. Scan converters (memories) store gray-scale image information and permit display on a television monitor. Analog scan converters store echo information as electric charge on a matrix of insulators. Digital scan converters are computer memories that store echo information as numbers in memory elements.

Exercises

5.6.1. The reflector information that can be obtained from an M-mode display includes

    a. distance and motion pattern

    b. transducer frequency, reflection coefficient, and distance

    c. acoustic impedances, attenuation, and motion pattern

    d. none of the above

5.6.2. The compensation (swept gain, etc.) control serves to

    a. compensate for machine instability in the warmup time

    b. compensate for attenuation

    c. compensate for transducer aging and the ambient light in the examining area

    d. decrease patient examination time

5.6.3. A gray-scale display shows

    a. gray color on a white background

    b. reflections with one brightness level

    c. a white color on a gray background

    d. a range of reflection amplitudes

5.6.4. The dynamic range of an ultrasound system is defined as

    a. the speed with which ultrasound examination can be performed

    b. the range over which the scanning arm can be manipulated while performing an examination

    c. the ratio of the maximum amplitude to the minimum amplitude or power that can be displayed

    d. the range of pulser voltages applied to the transducer

5.6.5. A digital scan converter is a _____ .

    a. compressor

    b. receiver

    c. display

    d. computer memory

    e. none of the above

5.6.6. Place the following in the order in which they are performed in a receiver:

    a. rejection

    b. amplification

    c. smoothing

    d. rectification

    e. compression

    f. compensation

5.6.7. Television displays produce _____ frames per second with _____ lines in each.

    a. 30, 60

    b. 30, 525

    c. 60, 512

    d. 512, 512

    e. 60, 120

5.6.8. In a digital instrument, echo intensity is represented by:

    a. positive charge distribution

    b. a number stored in memory

    c. electron density of the scan converter writing beam

    d. a and c

    e. all of the above

5.6.9. If there were no attenuation in tissue, _____ would not be
needed.
a. rejection
b. compression
c. demodulation
d. compensation

5.6.10. Devices called _____ send transducer location and
orientation information to the instrument.
a. scan converters
b. matching transformers
c. optical encoders
d. potentiometers
e. c and d

5.6.11. Which of the following are capable of displaying gray-scale
information?
a. storage CRT
b. television monitor
c. demodulator
d. a and b
e. none of the above

5.6.12. Reflection imaging includes ultrasound generation,
propagation and reflection in tissues, and reception of
returning _____ .

5.6.13. Virtually all the diagnostic ultrasound systems in use today
are of the _____ type.

5.6.14. Reflection-type instruments are also called
_____ instruments.

5.6.15. Reflection-type instruments look for three things: the
_____ , _____ , and
arrival _____ of reflections that occur in
tissues.

5.6.16. An analog scan converter stores image information in the
form of _____ .
a. electric charge
b. digital number
c. resistor temperature
d. impedence
e. none of the above

5.6.17. Imaging systems produce a visual _____
from the electric _____ received from the
transducer.

5.6.18. The transducer is connected to the memory through the
_____ .

5.6.19. The transducer receives voltages from the
_____ in pulse-echo systems.

5.6.20. The _____ receives voltages from the
transducer.

5.6.21. Increasing gain generally produces the same effect as
a. decreasing attenuation
b. increasing attenuation
c. increasing compression
d. increasing rectification
e. both b and c

5.6.22. Voltage pulses occur at the output of the
a. pulser
b. transducer
c. receiver
d. display
e. both a and b
f. both c and e

5.6.23. Ultrasound pulses from the pulser are applied to the
a. pulser
b. transducer
c. receiver
d. display

5.6.24. Rectification and smoothing are parts of
a. amplipression
b. rejection
c. a and b
d. compression
e. demodulation

5.6.25. If gain is reduced by one-half, and if input power is
unchanged, the output power is _____ what it was before.
a. equal to
b. twice
c. one-half
d. none of the above

5.6.26. If gain was 30 dB and output power is reduced by one-half,
the new gain is _____ dB.
a. 15
b. 60
c. 33
d. 27
e. none of the above

5.6.27. If four shades of gray are shown on a display, each twice the brightness of the next brightest one, the brightest shade is _____ times the brightness of the dimmest shade.

a. 2
b. 4
c. 8
d. 16
e. 32

5.6.28. The dynamic range displayed in Problem 5.6.27 is _____ dB.

a. 10
b. 9
c. 5
d. 2
e. 0

5.6.29. Gain and attenuation are usually given in

a. dB
b. dB/cm
c. cm
d. cm/3 dB
e. none of the above

5.6.30. Compensation (swept gain) makes up for the fact that reflections from deeper reflectors arrive at the transducer with greater amplitude. True or false?

Chapter 6

Dynamic Imaging Instruments

6.1 Introduction

Section 5.5 described how A-mode and M-mode presentations occur with the transducer held stationary. These presentations are one dimensional and **real-time** in nature. It was shown, however, that producing the two-dimensional images of the B scan required **scanning** the transducer. With such a manual static scanning process, it is not possible to produce images rapidly enough to produce a display that continuously images moving structures **(real-time display).**

Real-time or **dynamic imaging** instrumentation must produce several cross-sectional images per second. This requires the use of mechanical or array real-time transducers. Ten to 60 images are displayed per second **(frame rate),** yielding what appears to be a continuously changing image. Dynamic imaging instruments may or may not have a memory. Because the images are produced rapidly in sequence, memory is not required, as it is in the case of the manual scan, which takes a second or two to produce and then is observed for several seconds. If a real-time instrument has static-image (freeze-frame) capability, it must have a memory.

The advantages and disadvantages of static and dynamic systems are given in References 14–17. There are two primary advantages to real-time imaging:

1. more rapid and more convenient acquisition of the desired image
2. two-dimensional imaging of the motion of moving structures

112

The first advantage derives from the fact that the display continuously changes as the transducer is moved over the body surface. The second derives from the fact that the display continuously changes as the structures move.

There are two ways in which a dynamic B-mode display can be produced:

1. mechanical scan
2. electronic scan

Both of these methods provide a means for sweeping the sound beam through the tissues rapidly and repeatedly. The first method may be accomplished by oscillating a transducer in angle, rotating a transducer or a group of transducers, by oscillating a reflector, or by linearly translating a transducer. In most mechanical real-time transducers, the rotating or oscillating component is immersed in a coupling liquid within the transducer assembly. The sound beam is thus swept at a rapid rate without movement of the entire transducer assembly. Approaches to mechanical scanning are shown in Figure 6.1.

Electronic scanning is performed with arrays. **Transducer arrays** are transducer assemblies with several transducer elements. The elements are rectangular in shape and arranged in a line (**linear array**) or ring-shaped and arranged concentrically (**annular array**) (Figure 6.2).

A **linear switched array** (sometimes called a linear sequenced array or simply a linear array) is operated by applying voltage pulses to groups of elements in succession (Figure 6.3). Each group of elements acts like a larger transducer element in this case. The origin of the sound beam moves across the face of the transducer assembly and thus produces the same effect as manual linear scanning with a single-element transducer. Such electronic scanning, however, can be done in a more rapid and more consistent manner. If this electronic scanning is repeated rapidly enough, a real-time presentation of information can result. This requires scanning across the transducer assembly several times per second.

A **linear phased array** (commonly called a phased array) is operated by applying voltage pulses to all elements in the assembly as a complete group, but with small time differences, so that the resulting sound pulse may be shaped and steered (Figure 6.4). If the same time differences are used each time the process is repeated, the same beam shape and direction will result repeatedly. However, the time differences may be changed with each successive repetition, so that the beam shape (Figure 6.5) or direction (Figure 6.6) can continually change. This can then result in sweeping of the beam (the beam direction changes with each

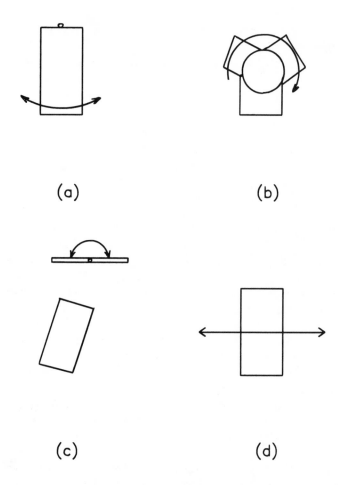

(a)

(b)

(c)

(d)

Figure 6.1. Mechanical real-time transducer types. (a) Oscillating transducer; (b) rotating group of transducers; (c) oscillating mirror (stationary transducer); (d) linearly translating transducer.

pulse) and in **variable focusing** (the focal length changes with each pulse).

A linear phased array can focus or steer electronically only in the scan plane (the vertical plane in Figure 6.4). Focus (fixed) can be achieved in the other plane with a lens. A linear array can be operated simultaneously as a switched and phased array, providing scanning, steering, and shaping of the beam. Annular phased arrays [Figure 6.2(b)] can focus in both planes but cannot provide beam steering. The addition of an oscillating mirror to these arrays provides a means for beam steering.

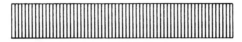

(a)

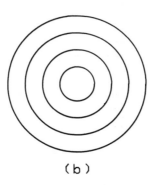

(b)

Figure 6.2. Front views of (a) a linear array with 64 rectangular elements and (b) an annular array with four elements.

When an array is receiving reflections, the electrical outputs of the elements can be timed so that the array "listens" in a particular direction with a listening focus at a particular depth. This received focus depth may be continually increased as the transmitted pulse travels through the tissues. This continually changing received focus is called **dynamic focusing.**

In addition to side lobes, which single-element transducers have (Section 4.3), arrays have **grating lobes,** which are additional beams resulting from their multi-element structure.

Exercises

6.2.1. Transducer arrays are transducer assemblies with more than one transducer _____ .

6.2.2. Two types of arrays are _____ and _____ .

6.2.3. Linear arrays are of two types according to how they are operated: linear _____ arrays and linear _____ arrays.

6.2.4. Match the following (answers may be used more than once):

    a. a linear switched array   1. scan
       can _____ the beam.   2. steer
    b. A linear switched array   3. shape
       cannot _____ or _____
       the beam.

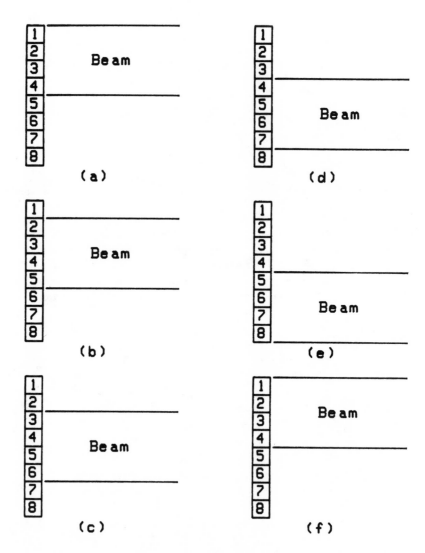

Figure 6.3. A linear switched array (side view). Voltage pulses are applied simultaneously to all elements in a group: (a) first to elements 1 through 4 as a group, (b) next to elements 2 through 5, and so on across the transducer assembly. Then the process is repeated (f).

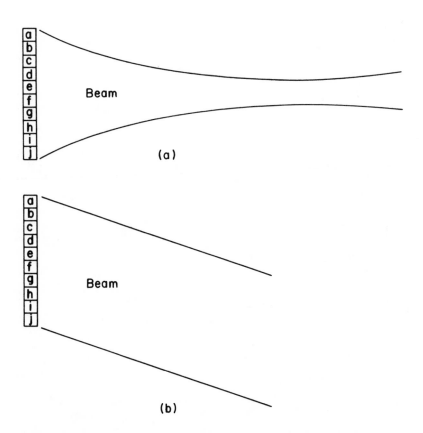

Figure 6.4. A linear phased array (side view). (a) By applying voltage pulses to the upper and lower elements earlier than to the middle elements, the beam can be focused. (b) By applying voltage pulses to the upper elements earlier than to the lower elements, the beam can be steered down. Similarly, by applying voltage pulses to the lower elements earlier, the beam can be steered up. Pulses may be applied in such a way that parts (a) and (b) are combined, resulting in a focused *and* steered beam.

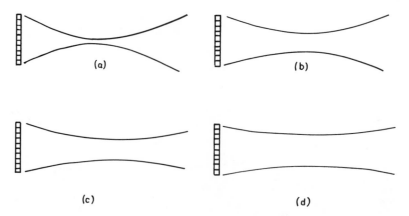

Figure 6.5. Variable focusing with a linear phased array. In the sequence (a) through (d), the time delays between applications of the electrical pulse to the elements are reduced. This results in weakening of the focus and a movement of the focus away from the transducer assembly. In some instruments, the delay can be controlled by the operator so that focal depth can be selected.

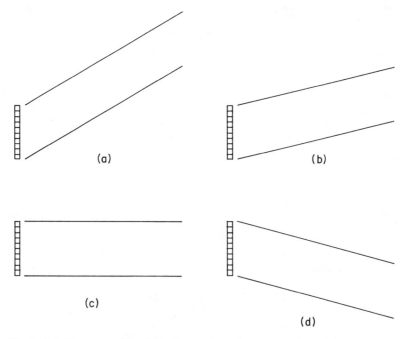

Figure 6.6. Beam steering with a linear phased array. (a) The pulse is directed at an upward angle because the voltage pulse from the instrument pulser is applied to the elements in rapid succession from bottom to top. (b) The next pulse travels out at less of an upward angle because the time delays in applying the voltage pulse to the elements are less than in (a). (c) The next pulse travels out horizontally because the voltage pulse is applied simultaneously to all the elements. (d) The next pulse is directed at a downward angle because the voltage pulse is applied in rapid succession to the elements from top to bottom.

    c. A linear phased array
       can _____ and _____
       the beam.
    d. An annular phased array
       can _____ the beam
       but cannot _____
       or _____ the beam.
    e. A combined linear switched
       and phased array can _____,
       _____, and _____
       the beam.

6.2.5. A linear array can scan, steer, or shape in _____ dimension(s).

6.2.6. An annular array can shape in _____ dimension(s).

6.2.7. An annular array can steer a beam with the aid of an

_____ / _____ .

6.2.8. Match the following (answers may be used more than once):

    a. linear switched
       array: _____
    b. linear phased array:
       _____
    c. annular phased
       array: _____

    1. Voltage pulses are applied in succession to groups of elements
    2. Voltage pulses are applied to all elements as a group, but with small time differences.

6.2.9. In Figure 6.4, if elements are pulsed in rapid succession in the order a, b, c, d, e, f, g, h, i, j, the resulting beam is
    a. steered up
    b. steered down
    c. focused

6.2.10. In Figure 6.4, if elements are pulsed in rapid succession in the order j, i, h, g, f, e, d, c, b, a, the resulting beam is
    a. steered up
    b. steered down
    c. focused

6.2.11. In Figure 6.4, if elements are pulsed in rapid succession in order a and j, b and i, c and h, d and g, e and f, the resulting beam is
    a. steered up
    b. steered down
    c. focused

6.3.
Real-Time Displays

Each complete scan of the sound beam produces an image on the display that is called a *frame*. Each frame is made of scan lines (one for each time the transducer is pulsed). The pulse repetition frequency is determined by the lines per frame and the frame rate:

pulse repetition frequency (Hz) = lines per frame × frame rate	PRF = LPF × FR

Two display formats result from the scanning methods described in the previous section: rectangular and sector (Figure 6.7). The linear mechanical transducer and the linear switched array produce a rectangular display. The oscillating and rotating mechanical transducers, the oscillating mirror, and the phased array produce a sector display format. In the rectangular format, the scan line density in the display is given in terms of lines per centimeter. This is determined by the lines per frame and the distance in centimeters represented by the width of the rectangular display.

line density (lines/cm) = $\dfrac{\text{lines per frame}}{\text{display width (cm)}}$	$LD = \dfrac{LPF}{Wd}$

For the sector scan format, the line density is determined by the number of lines per frame and the total sector angle (typically 45, 90, or 105 degrees).

line density (lines/degree) = $\dfrac{\text{lines per frame}}{\text{sector angle (degrees)}}$	$LD = \dfrac{LPF}{SA}$

Exercises

6.3.1. Match the following:

Real-time transducer	Display
a. linear mechanical _____	1. rectangular
b. oscillating _____	2. sector
c. rotating _____	
d. rotating mirror _____	
e. linear switched array _____	
f. linear phased array _____	

6.3.2. If the pulse repetition frequency of an instrument is 1 kHz and it displays 25 frames per second, there are _____ lines per frame.

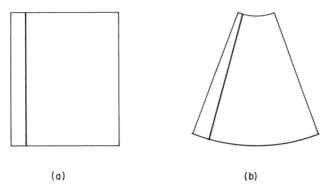

(a)   (b)

Figure 6.7. Rectangular (a) and sector (b) display formats for dynamic-imaging instruments.

6.3.3. The pulse repetition frequency is _____ Hz if there are 30 frames (40 lines each) per second.

6.3.4. If the instruments have rectangular displays with width representing 10 cm, the line densities for Problem 6.3.2 and 6.3.3 are _____ and _____ lines/cm, respectively.

6.3.5. If the instruments have sector displays representing 90 degrees, the line densities for Problem 6.3.2 and 6.3.3 are _____ and _____ lines/degree, respectively.

**6.4
Review**

Dynamic (real-time) imaging is the rapid sequential display of static ultrasound images resulting in a moving presentation. Such imaging requires rapid, repeatable, sequential scanning of the sound beam through the tissue. This is accomplished by mechanical real-time transducers of various types and by linear switched or phased transducer arrays. Rectangular or sector display formats result from such scanning techniques. Frame rates are typically 10 to 60 per second.

Exercises

6.4.1. The modes that show one-dimensional real-time images are the _____ mode and the _____ mode.

6.4.2. The mode that can show two-dimensional real-time images is the _____ mode.

6.4.3. A real-time B-mode display may be produced by rapid _____ transducer scanning or by _____ scanning of a transducer array.

6.4.4. Each complete scan of the sound beam produces an image on the display that is called a _____ .

6.4.5. The number of lines in each frame is equal to the number of times the transducer is _____ while the frame is produced (while the sound beam is scanned).

6.4.6. In real-time scanning, the pulse repetition frequency is equal to the number of _____ per frame times the _____ rate.

6.4.7 Real-time imaging permits imaging of the motion of moving structures, but it is not as convenient as static B-mode imaging for acquiring desired static images. True or false?

Chapter 7

Doppler Instruments

One item of information not used by the instruments described in Chapters 5 and 6 is the **Doppler shift** of the received reflections. Doppler instruments respond to moving reflectors or scatterers (usually blood cells in circulation) by detecting Doppler shift. This information is converted to audible sound or to a visual display. Doppler instruments are of two types:

1. continuous-wave Doppler instruments
2. pulsed instruments

Doppler instrument SATA intensities range from 0.2 to 400 mW/cm^2.

7.1. Introduction

In Chapter 3 only media boundaries that are stationary with respect to the sound source were considered. If a boundary is moving with respect to the source, the **Doppler effect** will occur. The Doppler effect is a change in reflected frequency caused by reflector motion. If the media boundary (reflector) is moving toward the source [Figure 7.1 (a)], the reflected frequency will be higher than the incident frequency. If the reflector is moving away from the source [Figure 7.1(b)], the reflected frequency will be lower than the incident frequency. The greater the speed of the boundary, the greater will be the difference between incident and reflected frequencies. The incident frequency subtracted from the reflected frequency is called the Doppler shift.

7.2 Doppler Effect

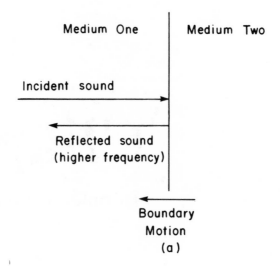

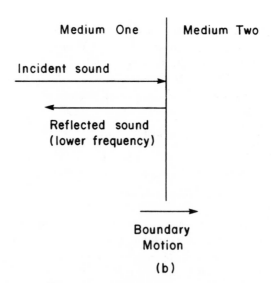

Figure 7.1. Doppler effect. (a) If the reflector (boundary) moves toward the source, the reflected frequency is higher than the incident frequency. (b) If the reflector moves away from the source, the reflected frequency is lower than the incident frequency.

Doppler shift (MHz) = reflected frequency (MHz) − incident frequency (MHz) = $\pm \dfrac{2 \times \text{reflector speed (m/s)} \times \text{incident frequency (MHz)}}{\text{propagation speed (m/s)}}$	$\begin{aligned} \Delta f &= f_r - f_i \\ &= \pm \dfrac{2 \times S_r \times f_i}{c} \end{aligned}$

The plus sign is used when the reflector is moving toward the source and the minus sign is used when the reflector is moving away from the source. If the direction of the incidence sound is not parallel to the direction of the boundary motion (Figure 7.2), the right side of the equation must be multiplied by the **cosine (cos)** (Appendix C) of the angle between these directions. Table 7.1 lists Doppler frequency shifts for several reflector or scatterer speeds. Table 7.2 gives examples of the effect of angle on Doppler shift. An instrument designed to measure the difference between the incident and reflected frequencies can yield information on reflector motion. The moving reflector could be a tissue boundary (e.g., a blood vessel wall or fetal heart) or a cell in suspension (e.g., blood cells in circulation). Commonly used frequencies are in the 2 to 10 MHz range.

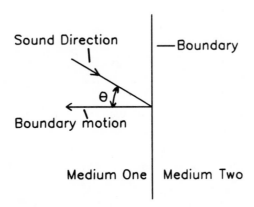

Figure 7.2. The Doppler shift depends on the angle, θ, between the direction of sound propagation and the direction of boundary (reflector or scatterer) motion.

Table 7.1.
Doppler Frequency Shifts for Various Scatterer Speeds
Toward the Sound Source*

Incident Frequency (MHz)	Scatterer Speed (cm/s)	Reflected Frequency (MHz)	Doppler Shift (kHz)
2	50	2.0013	1.3
5	50	5.0032	3.2
10	50	10.0065	6.5
2	200	2.0052	5.2
5	200	5.013	13
10	200	10.026	26

*Motion away from the source would yield negative Doppler shifts.

Exercises

7.2.1. The Doppler effect is a change in reflected
_____ caused by reflector
_____ .

7.2.2. If the reflector is moving toward the source, the reflected
frequency is _____ than the incident
frequency.

7.2.3. If the reflector is moving away from the source, the
reflected frequency is _____ than the
incident frequency.

7.2.4. If the reflector is stationary with respect to the source, the
reflected frequency is _____
_____ the incident frequency.

7.2.5. Measurement of Doppler shift yields information about
reflector _____ .

7.2.6. If the incident frequency is 1 MHz, the propagation speed is
1600 m/s, and the reflector speed is 16 m/s toward the
source, the Doppler shift is _____ MHz and the reflected
frequency is _____ MHz.

Table 7.2

Doppler Frequency Shifts for Various Angles and
Scatterer Speeds Toward the Sound Source of
Frequency 5 MHz

Scatterer Speed (cm/s)	Angle (°)	Doppler Shift (kHz)
100	0	6.5
100	30	5.6
100	60	3.2
100	90	0
300	0	19
300	30	17
300	60	9.7
300	90	0

7.2.7. If 2-MHz ultrasound is reflected from a soft-tissue boundary moving at 10 m/s toward the source, the Doppler shift is _____ MHz.

7.2.8. If 2-MHz ultrasound is reflected from a soft-tissue boundary moving at 10 m/s away from the source, the Doppler shift is _____ MHz.

7.2.9. Doppler shift is the difference between _____ and _____ frequencies.

7.2.10. When incident sound direction and reflector motion are not parallel, calculation of the reflected frequency involves the _____ of the angle between these directions.

7.2.11. If the angle between incident sound direction and reflector motion is 60 degrees, the Doppler shift and reflected frequency in Problem 7.2.6 are _____ MHz and _____ MHz.

7.2.12. If the angle between incident sound direction and reflector motion is 90 degrees, the cosine of the angle is _____ and the reflected frequency in problem 7.2.6 is _____ MHz.

Ultrasound Doppler instruments must provide continuous or pulsed voltages to the transducer and convert voltages received from the transducer to audible or visual information corresponding to reflector or scatterer motion. If an instrument can distinguish between positive and negative Doppler shifts, it is said to be **bidirectional.** Continuous-wave Doppler instruments consist of a continuous-wave voltage generator and a receiver that converts the change in frequency (Doppler shift) resulting from reflector or scatterer motion to an audible sound or to an image corresponding to the location of the moving objects.

A diagram of the components of a continuous-wave Doppler system is given in Figure 7.3. The voltage generator produces continuous voltage of frequency 2–10 MHz, which is applied to the source transducer. The ultrasound frequency is determined by the voltage generator. It is set to equal the operating frequency of the transducer (Section 4.2). In the transducer assembly there is a separate receiving transducer that produces a voltage with a frequency equal to the frequency of the reflected ultrasound. If there is reflector motion, the reflected ultrasound and the ultrasound produced by the source transducer will have dif-

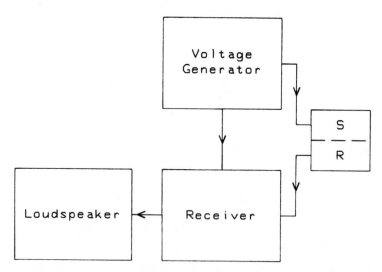

Figure 7.3. A continuous-wave Doppler instrument. The voltage generator produces a continuously alternating voltage that drives the source transducer (S). The receiving transducer (R) produces a continuous voltage in response to reflections it continuously receives. The receiver detects any difference in frequency between the voltages produced by the continuous-wave generator and by the receiving transducer. The Doppler shift produces a voltage that drives a loudspeaker in the audible range. The frequency of the audible sound is equal to the Doppler shift. It is proportional to the reflector speed and to the cosine of the angle between the sound propagation direction and the boundary motion (Section 7.2).

ferent frequencies. The receiver detects the difference between these two frequencies (the Doppler shift) and drives a loudspeaker at this difference frequency. The Doppler shift is typically one-thousandth of the source frequency, which puts it in the audible range.

If Doppler shift information is stored in memory at locations corresponding to anatomic sites of Doppler shift generation (motion), it may be presented as an image in addition to an audible sound. A block diagram of such an imaging instrument is given in Figure 7.4. The image is built up in memory as the transducer is scanned back and forth over the site of motion in the tissues. Only Doppler information is stored, so that the resulting image (Figure 7.5) represents an anatomic motion or flow map. Therefore, by using a scanning arm that sends information on transducer position to the electronics, a display can be produced that shows vessel anatomy along with pathology. This visual presentation can be enhanced by using color in a manner related to the Doppler shift. This improves the observer's ability to detect abnormal flow regions.

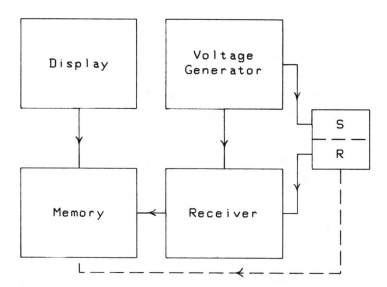

Figure 7.4. A continuous-wave Doppler imaging instrument. The operation is the same as in Figure 7.3 except that the output of the receiver goes to memory where Doppler shift information is stored at locations representing the skin surface locations where the reflections were received. Location information is sent from transducer-location sensors to the memory (dashed line). Memory output is sent to the display to present an anatomic image of motion (see Figure 7.5). For clarity, the loudspeaker is not included in this figure although it is a part of the instrument (as in Figure 7.3).

Transducer
Scanning
Motion

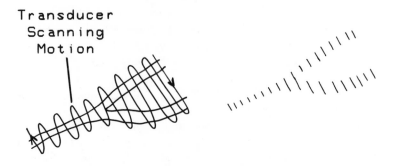

(a)   (b)

Figure 7.5. As the transducer is scanned back and forth across the skin over a vessel (a), Doppler shift information is stored in memory. Memory output to display produces a surface image (b) of motion or flow.

Exercises

7.3.1. All Doppler instruments distinguish between positive and negative Doppler shifts. True or false?

7.3.2. Instruments that distinguish between positive and negative Doppler shifts yield motion _____ information and are called _____ .

7.3.3. Continuous-wave Doppler instruments use single-element transducers similar to those used in static imaging. True or false?

7.3.4. The components of a cw Doppler system include _____

_____ ,

_____ _____ ,

_____ _____ ,

_____ , and _____ .

7.3.5. The frequency of the voltage from the receiver (representing the Doppler shift) must be converted to a frequency suitable for listening to the loudspeaker. True or false?

7.3.6. Scanning is not required for imaging with cw Doppler ultrasound. True or false?

7.3.7. Memory is not required for imaging with cw Doppler ultrasound. True or false?

7.3.8. A cw Doppler ultrasound image represents cross-sectional anatomy as sliced through tissue by the sound beam. True or false?

A diagram of the components of a pulsed Doppler instrument is given in Figure 7.6. The voltage generator is similar to that in Figure 7.3. The **generator gate** allows pulses of a few cycles of voltage to pass on to the transducer where ultrasound pulses are produced. The transducer assembly normally contains only one transducer element, which functions as both the source and receiving transducer. Voltage pulses resulting from received reflections are processed in the receiver. The frequency of the pulses is compared with the voltage generator frequency, and the Doppler shift is derived. It is sent to the loudspeaker for an audible output. Based on the arrival time of reflections (range

7.4 Pulsed Instruments

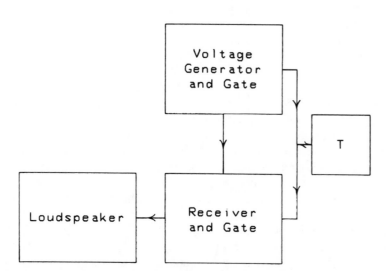

Figure 7.6. A pulsed Doppler instrument. The voltage generator produces a continuously alternating voltage. The generator gate converts this continuous voltage to voltage pulses that drive the transducer (T). This is normally a single-element transducer. Received pulses are delivered to the receiver, where their frequency is compared with the generator frequency. The difference (Doppler shift) is sent to the loudspeaker. The receiver also contains a gate that selects reflections from a given depth according to arrival time and thus gives motion information as a function of depth.

equation; Section 3.5), those coming from reflectors at a given depth may be selected by the **receiver gate;** thus, motion information may be obtained as a function of depth. Receiver gate width and location (depth into tissue) are controllable by the operator. There is an upper limit to Doppler shift that can be detected by pulsed instruments—approximately one-half the pulse repetition frequency (in the range of 5–30 kHz). Higher pulse repetition frequencies permit higher Doppler shifts to be detected but also increase the chance of range ambiguity artifact (see Chapter 8). Continuous-wave Doppler instruments do not have this limitation (but neither do they provide any depth information).

A single receiver gate selects one listening depth from which returning Doppler shifted echoes are accepted. The gate has some width (depth range) over which it permits reception. For example (using the range equation; 13 μs roundtrip travel time per centimeter of depth—Section 3.5), a gate that passes echoes arriving from 13 to 15 μs after pulse generation is effectively listening at a depth range of 10.0 to 11.6 mm. In this case the gate is located at a depth of 10.8 mm with a width (depth range) of plus or minus 0.8 mm. A single gate allows only one depth and width selection (from which all Doppler-shifted echoes will be accepted in combination) at any time. To simultaneously receive and separate Doppler information from several depths (e.g., to obtain a flow profile across a vessel) multiple gates must be used. These separate the Doppler information from several depths into separate channels for processing and display.

It is possible to obtain images with pulsed Doppler ultrasound in a manner similar to conventional pulse-echo imaging. The block diagram of a pulsed Doppler imaging instrument is given in Figure 7.7. The location of moving objects is determined by transducer location and orientation sensors and echo arrival timing as described for cross-sectional B-scanning in Chapter 5. This provides a cross-sectional image, in depth, of motion and flow in tissue. In Chapter 5, echo amplitude was displayed, while here Doppler shift is displayed. Thus, only moving reflectors or scatterers are imaged.

Combinations of instruments discussed in Chapter 6 and 7 are available commercially. Pulsed and cw Doppler systems are available in the same instrument. Real-time cross-sectional ultrasound imaging instruments are available with pulsed or cw and pulsed Doppler. These provide the capability of imaging anatomy as well as analyzing motion and flow at a known point in the anatomy (Figure 7.8). The availability of cw and pulsed Doppler in the same system is useful because difficulty is encountered in a pulsed system if the flow rates become so high that the Doppler shift approaches the pulse repetition frequency (discussed above). At that point the ability to shift to the cw system (even though it means giving up depth information) is advantageous.

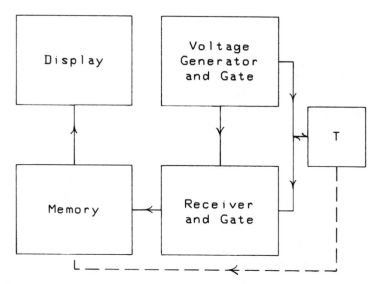

Figure 7.7. A pulsed Doppler imaging instrument. The operation is the same as in Figure 7.6 except that the output of the receiver goes to memory where Doppler shift information is stored at locations representing the anatomic locations of the moving reflectors or scatterers. This location information is obtained in the same way as in conventional cross-sectional B-scanning (Chapter 5). The difference here is that Doppler shift values are stored rather than echo-amplitude values. For clarity, the loudspeaker is not included in this figure although it is a part of the instrument (as in Figure 7.6).

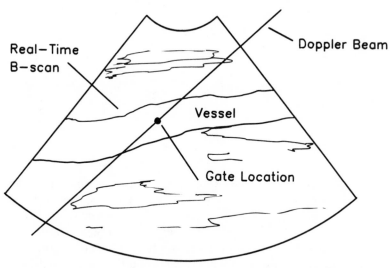

Figure 7.8. Image from a combined real-time and pulsed-Doppler instrument. The Doppler receiver gate depth can be located visually inside a vessel.

Exercises

7.4.1. The components of a pulsed Doppler instrument are the same as those for a cw instrument except for the addition of two _____ and the combining of two _____ into one.

7.4.2. The purpose of the generator gate is to convert a _____ voltage to a _____ voltage.

7.4.3. The purpose of the receiver gate is to allow selection of Doppler-shifted echoes from specific _____ according to _____ _____ .

7.4.4. Pulsed Doppler instruments require a two-element transducer assembly. True or false?

7.4.5. Multiple gates provide motion or flow _____ information.

7.4.6. The pulsed-Doppler imaging instrument gives a cross-sectional display of motion and flow as a function of depth in tissue. True or false?

7.4.7. There is no problem with interference of Doppler shifts with the pulse repetition frequency as long as the Doppler shifts are _____ half the pulse repetition frequency.
a. less than
b. equal to
c. greater than
d. all of the above
e. none of the above

7.4.8. To simultaneously receive and display Doppler information from several depths, several _____ must be used in the receiver.

7.5 Spectral Analysis

Because pulses sent into the tissues contain many frequencies in addition to the operating frequency of the transducer (Section 4.2) and because a distribution of flow velocities is encountered by the sound pulses as they traverse a vessel, a distribution of many Doppler-shifted frequencies returns to the transducer and the instrument (Figure 7.9). Since a presentation like Figure 7.9 is continuously changing with heart cycle, it can be displayed as a function of time with appropriate frequency spectrum processing (Figure 7.10). These displays provide quantitative data for evaluating Doppler-shifted echoes otherwise presented audibly or visually.

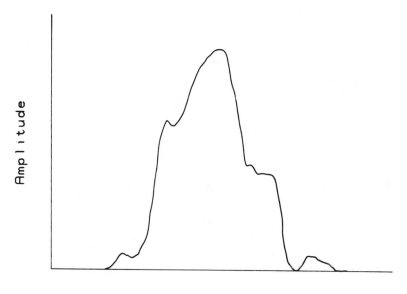

Figure 7.9. A frequency spectrum plot. This is a plot of the amplitude of each frequency component present in the returned pulse. Many frequencies are present because of the bandwidth of the transmitted pulse (Section 4.2) and the distribution of flow velocities encountered by the pulse in the gate region.

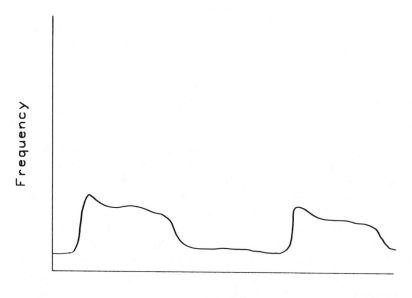

Figure 7.10. A display of spectrum as a function of time (heart cycle). Frequency is now on the vertical axis. The amplitude of each frequency component at each instant of time is represented by gray level or color.

7.5.1. Quantitative information about the frequencies contained in returning Doppler-shifted echoes can be displayed on an _____ versus _____ plot that is continuously changing with time.

7.5.2. To display the pattern of time change of a Doppler frequency spectrum, a display of _____ versus _____ can be used.

7.5.3. In Problem 7.5.2, the amplitude of each frequency component is represented by _____ level or

_____ .

7.5.4. The received frequency spectrum exists (rather than a single frequency) because of the _____ of the transmitted pulse and the distribution of

_____ _____

encountered by the pulse.

7.5.5. Since velocity is speed *and* direction, variations in either of these in the flow region interrogated by the Doppler instrument may contribute to the received frequency spectrum. True or false?

7.6 Review   The Doppler effect is a change in frequency resulting from reflector or scatterer motion toward or away from the source. Doppler instruments make use of this frequency shift to yield information regarding motion and flow. Continuous-wave systems provide motion and flow information without depth information or selection capability. Pulsed Dopplers provide depth information and the ability to select depth at which Doppler information is generated. Spectral analysis provides information on the distribution of received frequencies resulting from the bandwidth of transmitted pulses and the distribution of scatterer velocities encountered. In addition to audible output, imaging of vessel flow is possible in Doppler systems. Combined systems utilizing dynamic B-scan imaging and cw and pulsed Doppler are commercially available.

7.6.1. Doppler systems convert _____ _____ information to audible sound or visual display.

7.6.2 A pulser similar to that used in imaging systems is used in Doppler systems. True or false?

7.6.3 Doppler system transducers may have _____ or _____ elements.

7.6.4. The receiver in a Doppler system compares the _____ of the voltage generator and the voltage from the receiving transducer.

7.6.5. The Doppler *shift* usually is not in the audible frequency range and must be converted by the receiver to a frequency that can be heard. True or false?

7.6.6. Doppler shift is determined by reflector _____ and by the cosine of an angle.

7.6.7. A component that pulsed Doppler systems have but continuous-wave Doppler systems do not have is the _____ .

7.6.8. A Doppler system may have as an output a visual _____ .

7.6.9. In a pulsed Doppler system, the pulse repetition frequency is determined by the generator _____ , and the source ultrasound frequency is determined by the _____ _____ .

7.6.10. Pulsed Doppler systems can give motion information as a function of _____ .

7.6.11. A typical SATA output intensity for a Doppler instrument is 10 mW/cm^2. True or false?

7.6.12. The sound received by the transducer in a Doppler instrument is in the audible frequency range. True or false?

7.6.13. Frequencies used in Doppler ultrasound are in approximately the same range as those for pulse-echo imaging. True or false?

7.6.14. If the incident frequency is 4 MHz, the reflector speed is 100 cm/s, and the angle between beam and motion directions is 60 degrees, the Doppler shift is _____ kHz.

7.6.15. There is no problem in Exercise 7.6.14 with interaction of the Doppler shift with a pulse repetition frequency of 10 kHz. True or false?

7.6.16. If there were a problem in Exercise 7.6.15, _____ Doppler ultrasound could be used to avoid it.

Chapter 8

Artifacts

In imaging, an artifact is anything not properly indicative of the structures imaged. It is caused by some characteristic of the imaging technique. Because some artifacts are useful (e.g., **shadowing, enhancement,** speed error), imaging can at times be better than direct viewing of the anatomy (if it were possible). This is because some ultrasound imaging artifacts, although errors from an anatomic imaging standpoint, give valuable information on the nature of objects or lesions that might not be apparent with other imaging methods or even direct viewing. In addition to helpful artifacts, there are several that hinder proper interpretation and diagnosis. These must be avoided or properly handled when encountered.

8.1 Introduction

Artifacts in ultrasound imaging[18] occur as structures that are one of the following:

8.2 Artifacts

1. not real
2. missing
3. improperly located
4. of improper brightness
5. of improper shape
6. of improper size

Some artifacts are produced by improper equipment operation (e.g., improper transducer location and orientation information sent to the display) or settings (e.g., incorrect receiver compensation settings). Some are caused by improper scanning technique (e.g., allowing patient or organ movement during scanning). Others are inherent in the ultrasound diagnostic method and can occur even with proper equipment and technique.

Artifacts that occur in ultrasound imaging include:

resolution	grating lobe
texture	critical angle
slice thickness	multipath
reverberation	mirror image
curved reflector	shadowing
oblique reflector	enhancement
refraction	speed error
side lobe	range ambiguity

The assumptions in the design of ultrasound imaging instruments are that sound travels in straight lines, that the amplitude or intensity of returning echoes is related to the reflecting or scattering properties of distant objects, and that the distance to reflecting or scattering objects is proportional to the round trip travel time (13 microseconds per centimeter of depth).

Lateral and axial resolution limitations are artifactual in nature since a failure to resolve means a loss of detail and two adjacent structures may be visualized as one. Resolution was discussed in Section 4.4 in terms of separation of two reflectors (see Figures 4.13 and 4.14). If separation is not sufficient, two reflectors are seen as one (missing-reflector artifact). Resolution also increases the apparent size of a reflector on a display (Figure 8.1). The minimum displayed lateral and axial dimensions will be the beam diameter and one-half the spatial pulse length, respectively. Apparent image resolution can be deceiving. This is not directly related to tissue scattering properties (texture) but is a result of interference effects of the scattered sound from the distribution of scatterers in the tissue. This phenomenon is called acoustic speckle (see Section 3.4).

The beam width perpendicular to the scan plane results in slice thickness artifacts, for example, the appearance of false debris in echo-free areas and the presentation of cystic objects as being solid (e.g., gallbladder). This is because the interrogating beam has finite thickness as it scans through the patient. Echoes are received that originate not only from the center of the beam but also from the edges.

If two or more reflectors are encountered in the sound path, **multiple reflections (reverberations)** will occur. These may be sufficiently strong

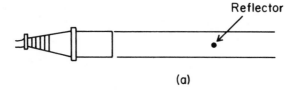

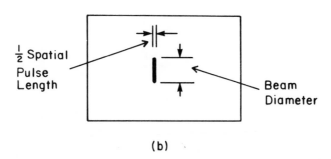

Figure 8.1. A tiny reflector (a) is displayed (b) with the axial dimension equal to one-half the spatial pulse length and the lateral dimension equal to the beam diameter. The image is produced by scanning the transducer from top to bottom in (a).

to be detected by the instrument and to cause confusion on the display. The process by which they are produced is shown in Figure 8.2. This results in reflectors that are not real being placed on the image. They will be placed behind the second real reflector at separation intervals equal to the separation between the first and second real reflectors (Figure 8.3). Each subsequent reflection is weaker than prior ones, but this will be at least partially compensated for by the compensation function of the receiver. The first reflector in Figures 8.2 and 8.3 is usually the transducer face.

Since diagnostic ultrasound is confined to beams (see Section 4.3), there are conditions in which all or part of the reflected sound may not return to the transducer and thus will be missed. Figures 8.4 and 8.5 show examples of simple situations in which this occurs. The **effective reflecting area,** the area that reflects sound *that is received* by the transducer, is smaller than the actual reflecting area in these cases. Therefore, reflector orientation and shape may reduce the amount of beam area received by the transducer. A curved reflector can produce a reflection low in amplitude because some of the reflection is missed by the transducer. Oblique reflection can produce a reflection low in amplitude, or the reflection may be completely missed by the transducer. This problem is reduced by reflector roughness, which adds

142

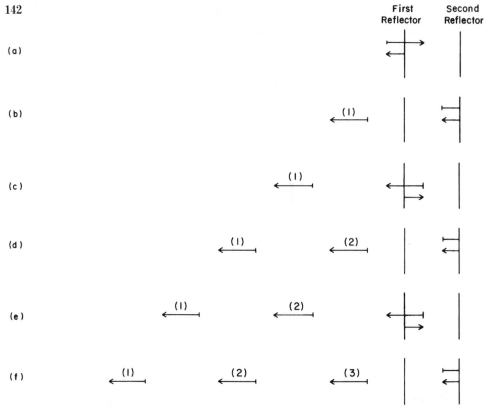

Figure 8.2. The generation of multiple reflections (reverberations). (a) An ultrasound pulse has come from the left, has encountered the first reflector, and has been partially reflected and partially transmitted. (b) Reflection and transmission at the first reflector are complete. Reflection at the second reflector is occurring. (c) Reflection at the second reflector is complete. Partial transmission (from right to left this time) and partial reflection are again occurring at the first reflector. (d) The reflections from the first (1) and second (2) reflectors are traveling to the left toward the sound source. A second reflection [repeat of (b)] is occurring at the second reflector. (e) Partial transmission and reflection are again occurring at the first reflector. (f) Three reflections are now traveling to the left: (1) is the reflection from the first reflector; (2) is the reflection from the second reflector; (3) is the reflection from the second reflector, reflected from the back side of the first reflector (c) and reflected again from the second reflector (d). A fourth reflection is being generated at the second reflector (f). Action proceeds from top to bottom in the figure.

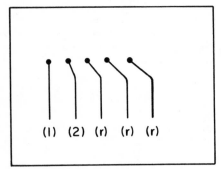

Figure 8.3. Reverberation on the display. (1) First real reflector (commonly the transducer face); (2) second real reflector; (r) reverberations. The separation between reverberations is the same as the separation between the real reflectors.

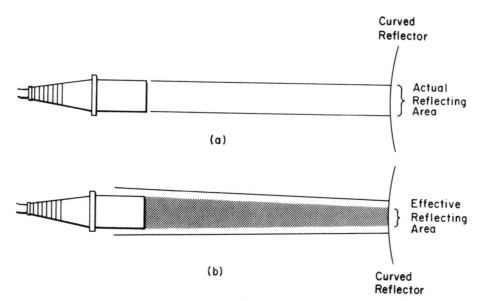

Figure 8.4. A curved reflector. (a) Incident sound on reflecting area. (b) Reflected sound from reflecting area. Only part of this reflected sound (shaded portion from the effective reflecting area) returns to the transducer. The remainder misses the transducer and continues on. The effective reflecting area is smaller than the actual reflecting area.

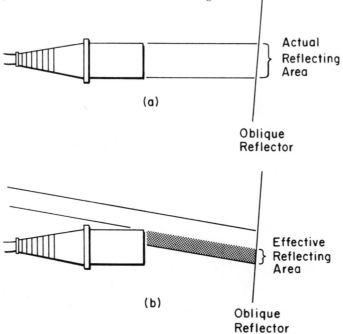

Figure 8.5. An oblique reflector. (a) Incident sound on reflecting area. (b) Reflected sound from reflecting area. Only part of this reflected sound (shaded portion) returns to the transducer from the effective reflecting area. The remainder misses the transducer and continues on. The effective reflecting area is smaller than the actual reflecting area.

143

backscatter to specular reflection. Increasing the frequency effectively increases the reflector roughness (see Section 3.4).

Refraction (see Section 3.3) can cause a reflector to be improperly positioned on the display (Figure 8.6). A similar occurrence can be caused by reflections from side lobes (see Section 4.3) or grating lobes (see Section 6.2) (Figure 8.7).

If the sound speed in the second medium is greater than in the first, and the incidence angle becomes large enough, the transmission angle reaches 90 degrees. The value of the incidence angle at this point is called the critical angle. At and beyond the critical angle, total reflection occurs (no transmission into the second medium). Thus, no imaging will occur beyond this boundary under this condition.

The term **multipath** describes the situation in which the paths to and from a reflector are different (Figure 8.8). Multipath results in improper reflector image positioning (increased range).

The mirror image artifact is the presentation of objects that are present on one side of a strong reflector on the other side as well (Figure 8.9). This commonly occurs around the diaphragm.

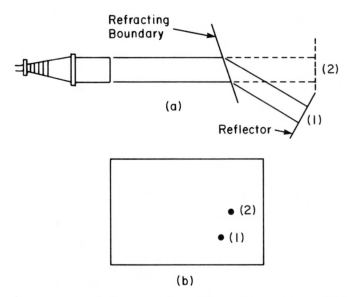

Figure 8.6. Improper positioning of the reflector on the display (b) because of refraction (a). The system thinks the reflector is at position 2 because that is the direction in which the transducer is pointing. The reflector is actually at position 1.

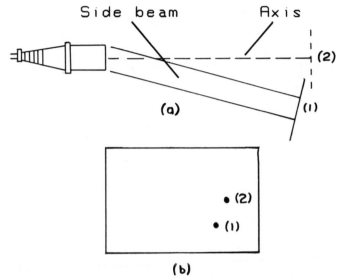

(a)

(b)

Figure 8.7. A side lobe or grating lobe can produce and receive a reflection from a "side view." This will be placed on the display at the proper distance from the transducer but in the wrong location (direction). This is because the instrument assumes that echoes originate from points along the transducer axis (the direction in which it is pointing). The instrument thinks that the reflector is at position 2 because that is the direction in which the transducer is pointing. The reflector is actually in position 1.

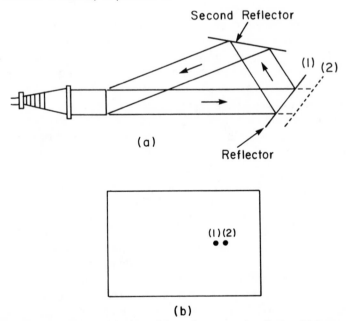

(a)

(b)

Figure 8.8. Improper positioning of the reflector on the display (b) because of multipath (a). The instrument thinks that the reflector is at position 2 because of the increased round-trip travel time required for a longer return path. The reflector is actually at position 1.

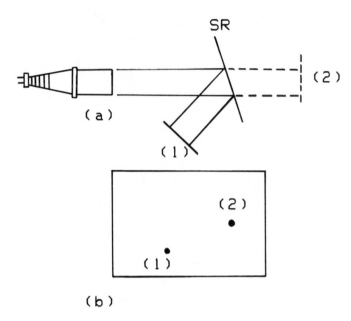

Figure 8.9. The mirror-image artifact occurs around strong reflectors (SR). The reflector that is located in position 1 is imaged in position 2 because that is the direction in which the transducer is pointing.

Shadowing is the reduction in reflection amplitude from reflectors that lie behind a strongly reflecting or attenuating structure. Enhancement is the increase in reflection amplitude from reflectors that lie behind a weakly attenuating structure. Shadowing and enhancement result in reflectors being placed on the image with amplitudes that are too low and too high, respectively. Shadowing and enhancement can also occur behind the edges of objects that are not necessarily strong or weak attenuators. In this case the cause is the focusing or defocusing action of a refracting curved surface. This increases or decreases the intensity of the beam beyond the surface, causing echoes to be strengthened or weakened. Shadowing and enhancement are useful artifacts for determining the nature of masses.

Propagation speed error occurs when the assumed value for propagation speed in the range equation (see Section 3.5) is incorrect. For diagnostic instruments a speed of 1.54 mm/μs is assumed. If the propagation speed that exists over a path traveled is greater than 1.54 mm/μs, the calculated distance to the reflector is too small, and the display will place the reflector too close to the transducer (Figure 8.10). If the actual speed is less than 1.54 mm/μs, the reflector will be displayed too far from the transducer. Refraction and propagation speed error can also cause a structure to be displayed with incorrect shape.

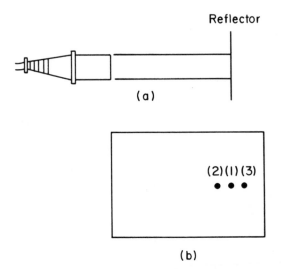

Figure 8.10. Reflector position on the display (b) depends on the propagation speed over the traveled path (a). The reflector is actually in position 1. If the actual propagation speed is less than that assumed, the reflector will appear in position 3. If the actual speed is more than that assumed, the reflector will appear in position 2.

In all of the operating modes discussed in Chapter 5, it is assumed that for each pulse, all reflections are received before the next pulse is sent out. If this were not the case, ambiguity could result (Figure 8.11). The maximum depth to be imaged unambiguously by an instrument determines its maximum pulse repetition frequency. The relationship between the two is:

maximum depth (cm) = 77/pulse repetition frequency (kHz)	$d_m = \dfrac{77}{PRF}$

In dynamic imaging, the pulse repetition frequency, the number of lines per frame, and the number of frames per second (frame rate) are related to one another (Chapter 6):

pulse repetition frequency (Hz) = lines per frame × frame rate	$PRF = LPF \times FR$

The relationship among lines per frame, frame rate, and maximum imaging depth in soft tissue is:

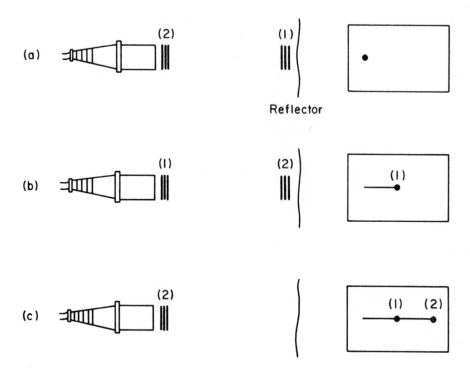

Figure 8.11. Ambiguity caused by sending out a pulse before a reflection from the previous pulse is received. (a) A pulse (2) is sent out just as a previous pulse (1) is reflected. (b) The spot begins to move across the display. The first reflection arrives at the transducer when the second pulse reflects. (c) The second reflection arrives at the transducer, putting a bright spot (2) on the display at the position corresponding to the reflector. The spot (1) in the center of the display resulting from the arrival of the earlier pulse indicates a reflector at a location where there is none.

maximum depth (cm) $\times$ lines per frame $\times$ frame rate = 77,000	$d_m \times$ LPF $\times$ FR = 77,000

For example, if the maximum imaging depth desired is 20 cm and the frame rate is 20 frames per second, there will be approximately 200 lines per frame maximum permitted to avoid ambiguity. If imaging at a greater depth is desired, either the frame rate or the lines per frame will have to be reduced.

The 77,000 comes from one-half the propagation speed in centimeters per second. Table 8.1 gives various values for pulse repetition frequency and maximum unambiguous imaging depth. These values apply to both static and dynamic imaging. Table 8.2 lists values of lines per frame, frame rate, and depth for dynamic imaging.

Table 8.1
Pulse Repetition Frequency (PRF) and
Maximum Unambiguous Depth to
Avoid Range Ambiguity

PRF (kHz)	Depth (cm)
7.7	10
3.8	20
2.6	30
1.0	77
2.0	38
3.0	26

Continuous-wave Doppler systems (see Section 7.3) can give motion artifacts if reflectors with different motions are included in the sound beam (e.g., two blood vessels being viewed simultaneously). Pulsed Doppler systems (see Section 7.4) help solve this problem by monitoring reflectors at selected distances or depths.

Table 8.2
Lines per Frame (LPF), Frames per Second
(Frame Rate: FR), and Maximum Depth to
Avoid Dynamic Imaging Range Ambiguity*

LPF	FR	Depth (cm)
1540	10	5
513	30	5
308	50	5
770	10	10
257	30	10
154	50	10
385	10	20
128	30	20
77	50	20

*LPF $\times$ FR = pulse repetition frequency (PRF in Table 8.1).

8.2.1. The maximum pulse repetition frequency that will unambiguously image to a maximum depth of 15 cm is _____ kHz.

8.2.2. The maximum depth for unambiguous imaging with an instrument having a pulse repetition frequency of 1 kHz is _____ cm.

8.2.3. If the propagation speed in a soft-tissue path is 1.60 mm/μs, a diagnostic instrument assumes a propagation speed too _____ and will show reflectors too, _____ the transducer.
   a. high, close to
   b. high, far from
   c. low, close to
   d. low, far from

8.2.4. Multipath can occur with only one reflector. True or false?

8.2.5. The minimum displayed axial dimension of a reflector is equal to
   a. beam diameter
   b. ½ × beam diameter
   c. 2 × beam diameter
   d. spatial pulse length
   e. ½ × spatial pulse length
   f. 2 × spatial pulse length

8.2.6. The minimum displayed lateral dimension of a reflector is approximately equal to
   a. beam diameter
   b. ½ × beam diameter
   c. 2 × beam diameter
   d. spatial pulse length
   e. ½ × spatial pulse length
   f. 2 × spatial pulse length

8.2.7. The fine texture in the region near the transducer indicates the extremely excellent resolution that actually exists in that region. True or false?

8.2.8. The fact that a beam, as it scans through tissue, has some finite width results in the _____ _____ artifact.

8.2.9. Which of the following can cause improper location of objects on a display? (More than one correct answer)
a. shadowing
b. enhancement
c. speed error
d. mirror image
e. refraction
f. side lobe

8.2.10. Refraction can cause shadowing. True or false?

8.3 Review

Axial resolution is determined by spatial pulse length. Lateral resolution is determined by beam width. Apparent resolution close to the transducer is not directly related to tissue texture but is a result of interference effects from a distribution of scatterers in the tissue. The beam width perpendicular to the scan plane results in slice thickness artifacts. Reverberation produces a set of equally spaced artifactual echoes distal to the real reflector. The mirror image artifact is the presentation of objects that are present on one side of a strong reflector, on the other side as well. Enhancement results from low attenuation objects in the sound path. Shadowing results from strongly reflecting or strongly attenuating objects in the sound path. Propagation speed error and refraction can cause objects to be displayed improperly in location and/or size or both. Refraction can also cause edge shadowing or enhancement.

Exercises

8.3.1. Match these artifact causes with their results:

a. reverberation: _____
b. shadowing: _____ ,

_____

c. enhancement: _____
d. curved reflector: _____
e. oblique reflector: _____ ,

_____

f. propagation speed error:

_____ , _____

g. refraction: _____ , _____
h. multipath: _____
i. resolution: _____ , _____

1. unreal structure displayed
2. structure missing on the display
3. structure displayed with improper brightness
4. improperly positioned structure
5. improperly shaped structure
6. structure of improper size

8.3.2. Reverberation results in added reflectors being imaged with equal _____ .

8.3.3. In reverberation, subsequent reflections are _____ than previous ones.

8.3.4. Enhancement is caused by a
a. strongly reflecting structure
b. weakly attenuating structure
c. strongly attenuating structure
d. refracting boundary
e. propagation speed error

8.3.5. A reflector may be missing from the display because of
a. reverberation
b. propagation speed error
c. enhancement
d. oblique reflection
e. Doppler shift
f. Snell's law

8.3.6. Shadowing results in decreased reflection amplitudes. True or false?

8.3.7. Propagation speed error results in improper _____ position of a reflector on the display.
a. lateral
b. axial

8.3.8. If the maximum depth imaged is 20 cm and the frame rate is 20 frames per second, there can be, at most, _____ lines per frame.

8.3.9. The pulse repetition frequency in Problem 8.3.8 is _____ kHz.

8.3.10. If there are 200 lines per frame and 25 frames per second, can 20 cm of depth be imaged unambiguously?

Chapter 9

Performance Measurements

9.1 Introduction

This chapter describes devices and methods used to determine if diagnostic ultrasound imaging instruments are operating correctly and consistently. These devices and methods are considered in three groups: (1) those that test the operation of the instrument as a whole (imaging performance); (2) those that measure the beams produced by transducers; and (3) those that measure the acoustic output of the instrument. Group 1 takes into account the operations of all the components shown in Figure 5.2. Group 2 considers only the transducer. Group 3 considers only the pulser and the transducer acting as a source. In group 2 tests, the transducer is driven and evaluated by a separate test generator or by the diagnostic instrument. Imaging performance is important for evaluating the instrument as a diagnostic tool. Beam profiles are important when evaluating and choosing transducers. The acoustic output of an instrument is important when considering bioeffects and safety (see Chapter 10).

9.2 Imaging Performance

Imaging performance is determined by measuring the following parameters:

1. relative system sensitivity
2. axial resolution (Section 4.4)
3. lateral resolution (Section 4.4)

4. **dead zone**
5. range (depth or distance) accuracy (see Sections 3.5 and 5.5)
6. **registration** accuracy
7. compensation (swept gain) operation (Section 5.3)
8. gray-scale dynamic range

These may all be measured using the 100-mm test object of the American Institute of Ultrasound in Medicine (AIUM) (Figure 9.1). This test object is composed of a series of 0.75-mm-diameter stainless-steel rods arranged in a pattern between two transparent plastic sides. The other sides are made of thin acrylic plastic sheets on which the transducer may be placed using a coupling medium. The tank is filled with a mixture of alcohol, algae inhibitor, and water that has a propagation speed of 1.54 mm/μs at room temperature. The speed varies by less than 1 percent when the temperature is changed by 5°C. Therefore, results with this test object are relatively insensitive to normal fluctuations in room temperature. Construction details and procedures for its use have been published.[19–21] These test objects are available commercially.

To obtain consistent measurements of axial and lateral resolution and dead zone, even with a given transducer and diagnostic instrument, it is necessary to perform the test at consistent control settings. Usually it is best to measure relative system sensitivity first and then increase the sensitivity settings a fixed amount for performing the other tests.

Relative system sensitivity is a measure of how weak a reflection an instrument can display. It is obtained by finding the gain or attenuation setting (with no compensation) at which a particular rod in the test

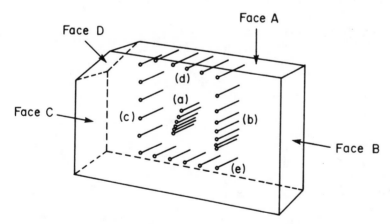

Figure 9.1. The AIUM 100-mm test object. Rod groups are used for measuring (a) axial resolution, (b) or (c) lateral resolution, (c) range accuracy and receiver compensation, (d) dead zone, and (a) through (e) registration accuracy. Any rod imaged may be used for sensitivity or dynamic range measurements.

object produces a barely discernible display. Any imaged rod may be chosen for this measurement. Usually the top rod in group (a) or the bottom rod in group (c) is used for system sensitivity measurements (Figure 9.1). For the remaining measurements, 10 dB are added to the system sensitivity settings required to barely display the chosen rod.

Axial resolution is measured with rod group (a). The transducer is placed on face A above the rod group. Not all the rods will be seen separately on the display. The spacing of the two closest rods in the group that are seen separately on the display is equal to the axial resolution (Figure 9.2). Axial resolution measured with the test object usually does not reflect the best possible resolution of the diagnostic system. The measurement, however, is a consistency check for use with a given transducer and instrument.

Lateral resolution is measured with rod group (b). The transducer is scanned along face B. Not all the rods will be seen separately on the display. The spacing of the two closest rods in the group that are seen separately on the display is equal to the lateral resolution [Figure 9.3 (a)]. Lateral resolution at a range from 1 to 11 cm can be determined by measuring the width of the line representing each rod in group (c) after the transducer is scanned across face A of the test object [Figure 9.3 (b)].

The dead zone is the distance closest to the transducer in which imaging cannot be performed. It is measured with rod group (d). The transducer is scanned across face A. The distance from the transducer to the first rod imaged is equal to the dead zone.

Range accuracy is measured with rod group (c). The rods should appear on the display at 1, 3, 5, 7, 9, and 11 cm from the transducer (Figure 9.4). Relative distances between the rods should be accurate to at least 2 mm or less. The space between the rods at 1 and 11 cm should be recorded with calipers and then measured with marker dots placed parallel to rod group (e). If this indicates that the distance be-

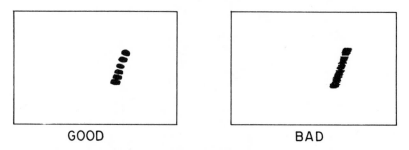

GOOD   BAD

Figure 9.2. Axial resolution. Rod group (a) in Figure 9.1 is used. Separations from 1 to 5 mm may be viewed. On the left, axial resolution is 1 or 2 mm. On the right it is 5 mm.

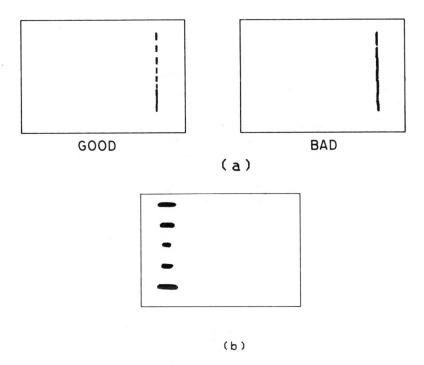

GOOD   BAD

(a)

(b)

Figure 9.3. Lateral resolution. (a) Using rod group (b) in Figure 9.1, separations from 3 to 25 mm may be viewed. On the left, lateral resolution is about 5 mm. On the right it is about 25 mm. (b) Using rod group (c) in Figure 9.1, the widths of rod images at various depths give lateral resolutions at these depths. A segmented picture of the beam is also presented with this view.

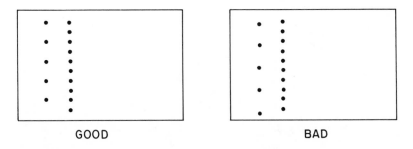

GOOD   BAD

Figure 9.4. Range accuracy is tested using rod group (c) in Figure 9.1. The rods should appear with 2-cm separations as on the left. One-centimeter marker dots are displayed here as well.

tween the rods at 1 and 11 cm differs from the true 10 cm by more than 2 mm, then the horizontal and vertical display scales are not identical.

Registration is the positioning of reflectors on the display. It depends on transmission of proper transducer location and orientation information, using the dash path from the transducer in Figure 5.2, and on satisfactory range accuracy, as described previously. Registration accuracy is measured using all the rods and scanning over faces A, B, C, and D. Correct registration results in star-shaped images at the location of each rod (Figure 9.5). Registration error is measured as the greatest separation between centers of any two lines in the image of any rod.[20]

Compensation operation is measured using rod group (c). The transducer is placed on face A above this rod group. With no compensation, the attenuator or gain settings required to display each rod at a given pulse height (A mode) or gray level (B or M mode) are recorded. This is then done again with compensation on. The difference between the settings for each rod as a function of distance is the compensation characteristic.

The gray-scale dynamic range is the difference between gain or attenuator settings (dB) that produce (1) barely discernible and (2) maximum deflection (A mode) or brightness (B or M mode) displays for the same reflection. Any rod imaged may be chosen for this measurement.

Several other objects are commercially available for testing imaging performance. These fall into two categories: test objects (e.g., the AIUM test object discussed above) and tissue-equivalent (TE) phantoms. Tissue-equivalent phantoms have some characteristics representative of tissues (e.g., scattering or attenuation properties) while test objects do not. Some objects are combinations of the two (e.g., an AIUM test object filled with tissue-equivalent medium rather than a water/alcohol

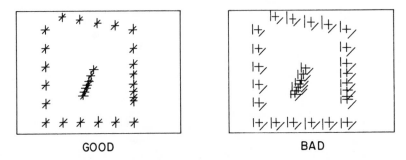

GOOD   BAD

Figure 9.5. Registration accuracy test. The star or asterisk presentation on the left indicates good registration.

mixture). The sensitivity, uniformity, and axial resolution (SUAR) test object uses a wedge cavity in a block to allow axial resolution measurement over a continuous range of separations. Tissue-equivalent phantoms containing echo-free (cystic) regions, scattering layers for scattered beam profile visualization, arrays of echo-free cylinders of various radii at various depths, cones containing material of various scattering strengths, or blocks of various scattering materials (gray scale levels) are available.

Exercises

9.2.1. The 100-mm test object contains several stainless-steel
_____ immersed in a mixture of algae
inhibitor, _____ , and
_____ that has a propagation speed 1.54
mm/μs.

9.2.2. Match the parameters measured with the rod groups used
(Figure 9.1) (answers may be used more than once):

a. axial resolution: _____   1. rod group (a)
b. lateral resolution: _____   2. rod group (b)
c. range accuracy: _____   3. rod group (c)
d. registration accuracy: _____   4. rod group (d)
e. dead zone: _____   5. rod group (e)
f. compensation: _____   6. all rods
g. sensitivity: _____   7. any rod
h. dynamic range: _____

9.2.3. Match the parameters measured with the types of
observation modes (answers may be used more than once):

a. axial resolution: _____   1. gain or attenuator settings
b. lateral resolution: _____   2. first rod imaged
c. range accuracy: _____   3. star-shaped images
d. registration accuracy: _____   4. rod distances from
e. dead zone: _____   transducer in the display
f. compensation: _____   5. minimum spacing
g. sensitivity: _____   of separately displayed rods
h. dynamic range: _____

9.2.4. Test objects are available commercially. True or false?

9.2.5. Results using a test object are relatively insensitive to
temperature. True or false?

9.2.6. The speed of sound in the recommended alcohol and water mixture of the AIUM test object varies by less than _____ percent when the temperature is changed by 5°C.

9.2.7. A limitation to the use of rod group (b) for lateral resolution measurement is that it yields an observation at only one _____ from the transducer.

9.2.8. To solve the difficulty in Problem 9.2.7, rod group (c) may be used to yield beam width information at several _____ .

9.2.9. Tissue-equivalent phantoms attempt to represent some acoustic property of _____ .

9.2.10. The AIUM test object is an example of a TE phantom. True or false?

9.3 Beam Profile and Frequency Spectrum

The test object described in Section 9.2 measures one beam parameter, the beam diameter, which is equal to lateral resolution. However, it does this only at one distance from the transducer: the distance from face B to rod group (b) in Figure 9.1. The use of rod group (c) in Figure 9.1 does not suffer from this same restriction. However, there is some distortion of the lateral resolution measurements in rod group (c) because of shadowing of lower rods by rods in the focal region. The test object is used to make this measurement using the ultrasound imaging instrument as a whole (the rod reflections are imaged on the instrument display). A **beam profiler** is a device designed to give three-dimensional reflection amplitude information. It uses a set of rods at various distances from the transducer (Figure 9.6). The transducer is pulsed as it is scanned across the tank. Reflections are received from each rod, and voltage amplitude is measured. As the sound beam passes over a rod, the reflected amplitude increases, goes through a maximum, and then decreases. Then the next rod (at a greater distance) is encountered, with a similar reflection behavior. This continues until all rods have been encountered. A beam profile can be plotted from this procedure (Figure 9.7). A beam profile does not actually give a profile of a beam, i.e., it does not plot acoustic amplitude or intensity across the beam at several distances from the transducer as it appears to do. It actually plots reflection amplitude received at the transducer, and it could be called a reflection profiler. For imaging instruments, however, this profile is a useful thing. Such profiles are often supplied with transducers to show beam characteristics obtained by this method. **Hydrophones** (see Section 9.4) can also be beam profilers in that they can measure pressure and intensity distributions across beams.

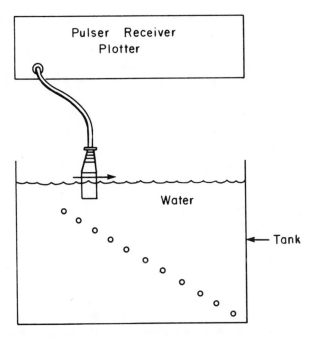

Figure 9.6. A beam profiler consists of a pulser, receiver, plotter, transducer, and tank with rods at various distances from the transducer. The transducer is scanned over the rods.

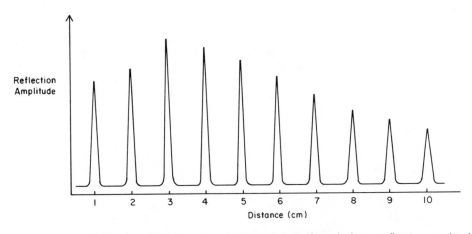

Figure 9.7. Beam profile plotted by the system in Figure 9.6. Each peak shows reflection amplitude as scanned across the rod that is at the distance indicated from the transducer. The amplitude is maximum at the near-zone length of an unfocused transducer or the focal region of a focused transducer (Section 4.3).

Two devices are commercially available that in a sense are beam profilers. One gives a beam cross section (perpendicular to propagation direction) that indicates intensity across the beam by liquid-crystal color changes. Another device provides a means to image the beam cross section on the gray-scale display of the diagnostic instrument. Gray-scale variations throughout the cross section indicate the degree of intensity nonuniformity across the beam.

Pulses produced by ultrasound transducers contain a range of frequencies called the bandwidth (Section 4.2). Transducer specifications often include a picture of the frequency spectrum of the pulses produced. This is a plot of amplitude (of each frequency component) versus frequency (Figure 4.6). It is obtained by receiving the pulse with a hydrophone (see Section 9.4) or with the same transducer that produced it (after reflection from a sphere, rod, or plate). The electric pulse from the hydrophone or transducer is sent to a spectrum analyzer, which breaks it down into its component frequencies and displays them as described above.

Exercises

9.3.1. Which of these devices measure(s) parameters related to beam profiling?
   a. 100-mm test object
   b. SUAR test object
   c. hydrophone
   d. both a and c
   e. both b and c

9.3.2. Reflection profilers plot acoustic amplitude or intensity across the beam at several distances from the transducer. True or false?

9.3.3. The following are often supplied with beam profiles to show their characteristics:
   a. pulsers
   b. transducers
   c. receivers
   d. displays
   e. both a and c

9.3.4. A spectrum analyzer is used to determine _____ .
   a. color spectrum
   b. impedance spectrum
   c. lateral resolution
   d. frequency spectrum
   e. all of the above

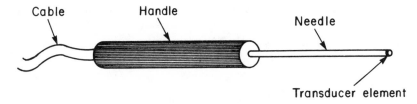

Cable   Handle   Needle   Transducer element

Figure 9.8. A hydrophone consists of a small transducer element mounted on the end of a needle.

Several devices can measure the acoustic output of ultrasound imaging instruments. Only one, the **hydrophone,** will be discussed here. The hydrophone is a small (1-mm diameter or less) transducer element mounted on the end of a narrow tube or hollow needle (Figure 9.8). Its size causes it to receive sound reasonably well from all directions without altering the sound by its presence. In response to the varying pressure of the sound, it produces a varying voltage that can be displayed on an oscilloscope. A picture similar to that in Figure 2.12 is produced, from which period, pulse repetition period, and pulse duration can be determined. From these quantities, frequency, pulse repetition frequency, and duty factor can be calculated. If the hydrophone calibration is known (relationship between voltage produced and pressure applied), pressure amplitude may also be determined. If propagation speed is known, wavelength and spatial pulse length can be calculated (Sections 2.2 and 2.3). If impedance is known, intensity can be calculated. Hydrophones are commercially available and are relatively inexpensive and simple to use.

**9.4
Acoustic
Output**

Exercises

9.4.1. Using a hydrophone, which of the following can be measured or calculated? (More than one correct answer)
a. impedance
b. amplitude
c. period
d. pulse duration
e. pulse repetition period

9.4.2. Hydrophones are commercially available and are relatively simple to use. True or false?

9.4.3. A hydrophone contains a small _____ element.

9.4.4. Because of its small size, a hydrophone can measure spatial details of a sound beam. True or false?

9.4.5. A hydrophone _____ .
a. interacts with light
b. produces a voltage
c. measures intensity directly
d. measures total energy
e. none of the above

9.4.6. Match the following (A can be calculated from B if C is known) (answers may be used more than once):

A:
a. frequency: _____ , _____
b. pulse repetition frequency: _____ , _____
c. duty factor: _____ , _____
d. wavelength: _____ , _____
e. spatial pulse length: _____ , _____
f. power: _____ , _____
g. intensity: _____ , _____

B:	C:
1. wavelength	7. number of cycles in the pulse
2. period	8. pulse duration
3. pulse repetition period	9. propagation speed
4. frequency	10. exposure time
5. energy	11. beam area
6. power	12. nothing else

9.5
Review

The 100-mm test object provides a means of measuring axial and lateral resolution, range and registration accuracy, dead zone, compensation, sensitivity, and dynamic range of diagnostic instruments. Beam profilers measure characteristics of beams produced by transducers. Hydrophones are used to measure the acoustic output of diagnostic instruments.

Exercises

9.5.1. Match these devices or phenomena with what they measure (answers may be used more than once):
a. beam profiler: _____
b. 100-mm test object: _____ , _____
c. hydrophone: _____ , _____

1. diagnostic instrument imaging performance
2. transducer beam characteristics
3. diagnostic instrument acoustic output

9.5.2. Match the following with the components about which they usually provide information:

a. hydrophone: _____
b. beam profiler: _____
c. 100-mm test
   object: _____

1. diagnostic instrument as a whole
2. pulser and transducer
3. transducer
4. transducer and receiver
5. receiver and display

Chapter 10

Bioeffects and Safety

10.1
Introduction

The interaction between ultrasound and tissues is pictured in Figure 1.1. The acoustic propagation properties of the interaction were discussed in Chapters 2 and 3. The bioeffects will be discussed in this chapter. Bioeffects are useful in therapeutic applications of ultrasound; that subject will not be considered here. Of concern is what the bioeffects of ultrasound tell us about the safety or hazard of the diagnostic ultrasound method. What would be desirable would be to ask the question, "Is it safe?" and to give the answer, "Yes." If this were possible, a separate chapter on the subject would not be needed. This ideal situation is not necessary for the procedure to be useful. Such a strong criterion is not applied to other areas of life. It cannot be said that riding in a car is safe; yet we choose to go off in one daily. What is desirable is knowledge of the probability of damage or injury and under what conditions this probability is maximized (in order to avoid those conditions) and minimized (in order to seek those conditions). In any diagnostic test there may be some risk (some probability of damage or injury). For diagnostic ultrasound, the sonologist and sonographer need to know something about this risk. Risk can be weighed against benefit to determine the appropriateness of the diagnostic procedure (Figure 10.1). Knowledge of how to minimize the risk is useful to everyone involved in diagnostic ultrasound.

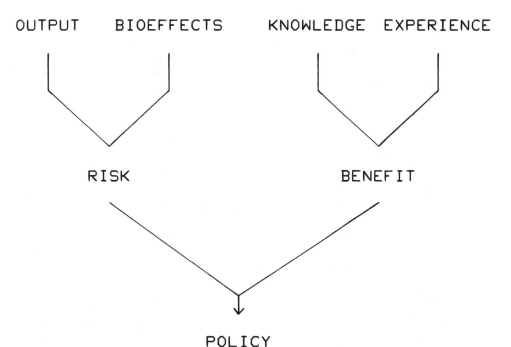

OUTPUT   BIOEFFECTS   KNOWLEDGE EXPERIENCE

RISK   BENEFIT

POLICY

Figure 10.1. Ultrasound risk and benefit information. Risk information comes from experimental bioeffects, epidemiology, and instrument output data. Benefit information comes from knowledge and experience in ultrasound imaging use and efficacy. Together they lead to policy on the prudent use of ultrasound imaging in medicine.

There are several sources of bioeffects information (Figure 10.2). However, a complete knowledge of the bioeffects of ultrasound is unavailable. What types of injury can diagnostic ultrasound produce in patients? Under what conditions? Sufficient epidemiologic data are not available.[22,23]

What is known is something about bioeffects in experimental animals. Hundreds of reports on this subject have appeared in the scientific literature. Several reviews of this subject have appeared.[22-26]

The Biological Effects Committee of the American Institute of Ultrasound in Medicine (AIUM) has reviewed the reports of bioeffects of ultrasound and has formulated the following statement[27-28]:

**10.2
Bioeffects**

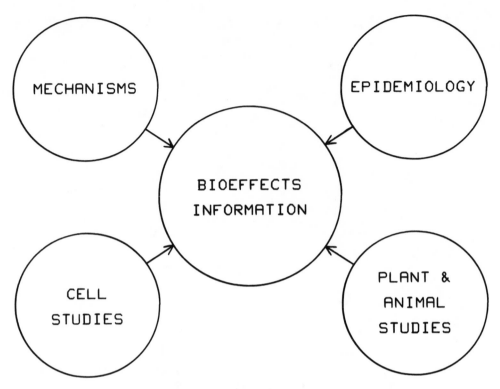

Figure 10.2. Bioeffects information sources.

Statement on Mammalian In Vivo Ultrasonic Biological Effects
Reaffirmed October 1982

In the low megahertz frequency range there have been no independently confirmed significant biological effects in mammalian tissues exposed to intensities* below 100 mW/cm². Furthermore, for ultrasonic exposure times** less than 500 seconds and greater than one second, such effects have not been demonstrated even at higher intensities, when the product of intensity* and exposure time** is less than 50 joules/cm².

*Spatial peak, temporal average as measured in a free field in water.
**Total time; this includes off-time as well as on-time for a repeated-pulse regime.

The low-megahertz range referred to in this statement is 0.5–10 MHz. The intensity considered is the SPTA intensity discussed in Section 2.4. "Measured in a free field" means that there were no reflections from the walls of the measuring system. "Repeated-pulse regime" (pulsed ultrasound) is discussed in Section 2.3. The product of intensity and time is intensity × time

$$= \left[\frac{power}{area} \right] \times \left[time \right] \qquad \text{(Section 2.4)}$$

$$= \left[\frac{energy}{time} \right] \times \left[\frac{time}{area} \right] \qquad \text{(Appendix D)}$$

$$= \frac{energy}{area} \; (\text{J/cm}^2) \qquad \text{(Table C.4)}$$

This is the energy passed through an area divided by the area.

This statement describes intensity and time limits below which "independently confirmed significant" bioeffects have not been reported. These limits are shown in Figure 10.3. They are probably not minimum or threshold levels. As more sensitive biologic end points are studied, it is reasonable to expect some lowering of these levels.

Reports used in determining the preceding statement considered the following bioeffects (see Section 5.2 of Nyborg[25]): hind-limb paralysis, fetal weight reduction, postpartum mortality, and liver mitotic index

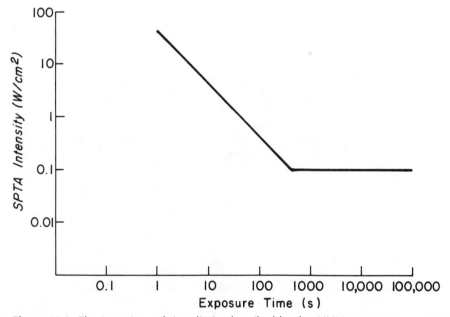

Figure 10.3. The intensity and time limits described by the AIUM statement on mammalian in vivo ultrasound bioeffects. There are no independently confirmed significant bioeffects in mammalian tissues for intensity and time conditions below the line. Intensity is SPTA as measured in a free field in water. Time is total time of exposure to ultrasound (includes time between pulses in the case of pulsed ultrasound).

reduction, all in mice and rats; blood vessel damage in chick embryos; wound healing in rabbit ears; postulated human fetal abnormalities based on absorption heating. The results were obtained with focused as well as unfocused beams, generated continuously or (to a lesser extent) as pulsed ultrasound.

A comparison of the instrument output data from Table 5.2 with the bioeffects statement levels is given in Figure 10.4. In making this comparison, the pulsed ultrasound of the instruments is compared with the continuous sound used in most bioeffects studies. This is done by using the SPTA intensity (see Section 2.4) of the pulsed ultrasound. If bioeffects depend on temporal average intensity, this is a valid comparison.

Three mechanisms of action for ultrasound bioeffects are generally recognized:

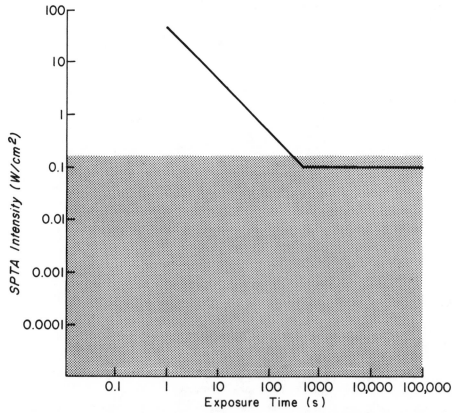

Figure 10.4. A comparison of instrument output data with the AIUM bioeffects statement level. The shaded area shows the range in which diagnostic instruments fall (Table 5.2). The SPTA intensity is used, assuming that temporal average is relevant. Time is total time of exposure to ultrasound (includes time between pulses in the case of pulsed ultrasound).

1. heat

2. **cavitation**

3. other

The third class is sometimes called mechanical. Little is known about it. For purposes here, it really means nonthermal and noncavitational. Heating depends on temporal average intensity. Cavitation does not. The intensity dependence of the category "other" is unknown.

The overlap in Figure 10.4 suggests that with the instruments that operate at the higher intensities, it may be possible to produce some bioeffects in small animals.

Another means of comparison is shown in Figure 10.5, where the SPTP intensity range of Table 5.2 is used. This assumes that individual pulses (typically 2–3 cycles long) can produce a bioeffect, that they add up (repair or recovery between pulses does not occur), and thus that bioeffects depend on temporal peak intensity. Whether or not any of this is true under any conditions is not currently known. If it were true, the overlap in Figure 10.5 would indicate that times greater than 1–50 s (depending on the SPTP intensity of the instrument) could pro-

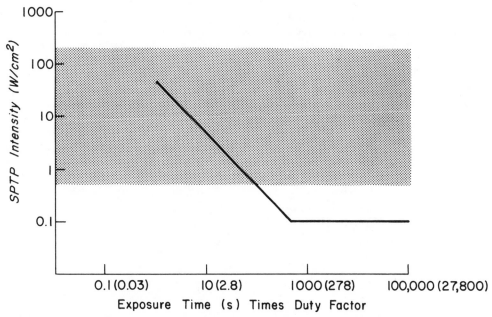

Figure 10.5. A comparison of instrument data with the AIUM bioeffects statement level. SPTP intensity is used (for pulsed ultrasound), assuming that temporal peak is relevant. The shaded area shows the range in which diagnostic instruments fall (Table 5.2). Time is sound-on time (total exposure time multiplied by duty factor for pulsed ultrasound). Exposure time in hours (assuming that the duty factor is 0.001) is given in parentheses.

duce bioeffects in animals. In this case, the appropriate time is the sound-on time, which is total exposure time multiplied by duty factor (typically 0.001). Total exposure times corresponding to 1–50 s sound-on time are (assuming a duty factor of 0.001) 1000–50,000 s (17 min to 14 h).

Another consideration in these comparisons is whether or not sound exposures separated by several hours or days add up (repair or recovery does not occur between exposures). No data are available to permit any statement on this consideration.

Several reports have appeared in the literature that appear to violate the AIUM statement. They do not, however, either because they do not deal with mammalian tissues or because they have not been independently confirmed. Several of these reports have dealt with in vitro studies. The relevance of these to clinical imaging safety is weak, at best. This is described by the AIUM Statement on in vitro Biological Effects (October 1982).[29]

Statement on In Vitro Biological Effects

It is often difficult to evaluate reports of ultrasonically induced in vitro biological effects with respect to their clinical significance. The predominant physical and biological interactions and mechanisms involved in an in vitro effect may not pertain to the in vivo situation. Nevertheless, an in vitro effect must be regarded as a real biological effect.

Results from in vitro experiments suggest new endpoints and serve as a basis for design of in vivo experiments. In vitro studies provide the capability to control experimental variables and thus offer a means to explore and evaluate specific mechanisms. Although they may have limited applicability to in vivo biological effects, such studies can disclose fundamental intercellular or intracellular interactions.

While it is valid for authors to place their results in context and to suggest further relevant investigations, reports that do more than that should be viewed with caution.

The AIUM Biological Effects Committee continuously reviews published articles relevant to ultrasound safety and publishes short critiques in the *Journal of Ultrasound in Medicine* (*Reflections* section). A compendium of these critiques is available.[30]

**10.3
Safety**

For consideration of the safety of diagnostic ultrasound, an attempt must be made to relate knowledge of bioeffects to the clinical situation (Figure 10.6). There are three questions that arise when an attempt is made to accomplish this:

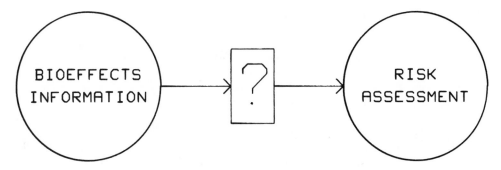

Figure 10.6. Relating bioeffects information to risk determination. Unanswered questions limit our ability to determine the relationship thoroughly.

1. Do any of the bioeffects that have occurred under experimental conditions constitute a hazard to a human in the clinical setting?
2. Are the acoustic parameters at the site of the bioeffect in experimental animals comparable to those at the appropriate site of concern in the body during diagnosis?
3. Do the continuous-wave conditions of most experimental studies provide any useful information for the pulsed ultrasound of clinical diagnosis?

These questions remain largely unanswered. Being unable to give a satisfying response to question 1, an attempt must be made to determine if *any* bioeffects observed in experimental animals are likely to occur clinically. This brings us to the difficulties of questions 2 and 3. The response to question 2 is that in human applications of ultrasound, the organs of concern are normally farther from the sound source (a longer attenuating sound path is involved). Also, a smaller organ volume fraction is exposed because the organs are larger than those of the experimental animals. Experimental studies are normally done with a stationary sound beam, whereas diagnostic studies usually involve scanning. These considerations may provide some (unknown) safety factors for the diagnostic situation. Question 3 was considered in the discussion of Figure 10.5.

Because a complete knowledge of bioeffects is unavailable, a conservative approach to safety considerations must be taken. *Use diagnostic ultrasound in an appropriate manner when benefit is expected from the procedure.* What constitutes "appropriate manner"? The following is quoted from an AIUM brochure on the subject[31]:

Diagnostic ultrasound has proven to be a valuable tool in medical practice and should be used without hesitation, with appropriate equipment and procedures, when medical benefit is expected. An excellent safety record exists in that after decades of clinical use there is no known instance of human injury due to diagnostic ultrasound.

Users should be aware of the factors related to ultrasonic exposure levels and should give serious consideration to intensity data when comparing various instruments. Other factors such as imaging quality, convenience, etc., are important, but if various instruments are equivalent in these aspects, the instrument with the lowest intensity levels should be favored. Increasing numbers of manufacturers are supplying intensity data for their equipment. The AIUM encourages the release of these data. Any manufacturer displaying the AIUM Manufacturer's Commendation Award for a specified model has satisfied AIUM requirements for determining exposure data for that model and for making the information publicly available.

It is important that users understand how they can minimize exposures in obtaining needed diagnostic information. Obviously, the shorter the examination, the less is the total exposure to the patient. In some equipment, controls are available which adjust the excitation of the transducer and change the emitted peak intensity or pulse repetition frequency. Different types of transducers can also exhibit different emitted intensity levels.

In assessing risk, overly simplistic attitudes should be avoided. The SPTA intensity of 100 mW/cm^2 should not be treated as a magic number. Levels under this value do not guarantee "perfect" safety, and levels above this value may well be appropriate if they are needed to yield diagnostic information. In choosing procedures and equipment, the obligation is always present to balance benefit against risk.

In short, we should minimize (unknown, but potentially non-zero) risk by minimizing exposure (Figure 10.7).

The AIUM has issued a safety standard[32] [in cooperation with the National Electrical Manufacturers' Association (NEMA)] and two statements[33-34] (March and October 1983) dealing with safety of diagnostic ultrasound in clinical care, education, and research.

Statement on Clinical Safety

Diagnostic ultrasound has been in use for over 25 years. Given its known benefits and recognized efficacy for medical diagnosis, including use during human pregnancy, the American Institute of Ultrasound in Medicine herein addresses the clinical safety of such use:

No confirmed biological effects on patients or instrument operators caused by exposures at intensities typical of present diagnostic instruments have ever been reported. Although the possibility exists that such biological effects may be identified in the future, current data indicate that the benefits to patients of the prudent use of diagnostic ultrasound outweigh the risks, if any, that may be present.

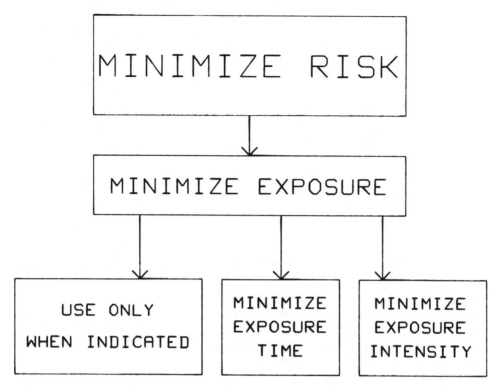

Figure 10.7. Minimize risk by minimizing exposure.

Safety Statement for Training and Research

Diagnostic ultrasound has been in use for over 25 years. No confirmed adverse biologic effects on patients or instrument operators caused by exposure at intensities and exposure conditions typical of present diagnostic instrument and examination practices have ever been reported. Experience from normal diagnostic practice may or may not be relevant to extended exposure times and altered exposure conditions. At this time, no hazard has been identified that would preclude the prudent and conservative use of diagnostic ultrasound in education and research.

The AIUM has stated that there have been no independently confirmed significant bioeffects in mammalian tissues exposed to SPTA intensities below 100 mW/cm². This indicates that with some instruments that operate at the higher intensities, it may be possible to produce some bioeffects in small animals. Whether or not they can occur in humans

**10.4
Review**

175

is unknown. Because there is limited specific knowledge, the conservative approach is taken: use diagnostic ultrasound with minimum exposure when benefit is expected from the procedure.

Exercises

10.4.1. There is no possible hazard involved in the diagnostic use of ultrasound. True or false?

10.4.2. Ultrasound should not be used as a diagnostic tool because of the bioeffects it can produce. True or false?

10.4.3. No independently confirmed significant bioeffects in mammalian tissues have been reported at intensities below
a. 10 W/cm^2 SPTP
b. 100 mW/cm^2 SPTA
c. 10 mW/cm^2 SPTA
d. 10 mW/cm^2 SATA
e. 1 mW/cm^2 SATP

10.4.4. Is there any knowledge of what types of injuries or risks occur with diagnostic ultrasound in patients, and under what conditions? Yes or no?

10.4.5. Is there any knowledge of any bioeffects that ultrasound produces in small animals under experimental conditions? Yes or no?

10.4.6. Heating depends most directly on
a. SATA intensity
b. SATP intensity
c. SPTP intensity

10.4.7. When SPTA intensities of pulsed and continuous-wave ultrasound are compared, the appropriate time to be used is
a. the total exposure time
b. the sound-on time

10.4.8. When SPTP intensity of pulsed ultrasound is compared with SPTA intensity of continuous-wave ultrasound, the appropriate time to be used is
a. the total exposure time
b. the sound-on time

10.4.9. The sound-on time is the total time multiplied by
a. beam uniformity ratio
b. pulse repetition frequency
c. Doppler shift
d. reflection coefficient
e. duty factor

10.4.10. The available epidemiologic data are sufficient to make a final judgment on the safety of diagnostic ultrasound. True or false?

10.4.11. Exposure is minimized by using diagnostic ultrasound
   a. only when indicated
   b. with minimum intensity
   c. with minimum time
   d. all of the above
   e. none of the above

Chapter 11

Misconceptions and Errors

11.1
Literature
Errors Misconceptions and errors regarding physical principles of diagnostic ultrasound regularly occur in the literature and in oral presentations. This indicates a lack of understanding of the physical principles of diagnostic ultrasound on the part of many in this field.

The inclusion of physical principles in the physicians' syllabus of The American Institute of Ultrasound in Medicine, the sonographers' syllabus of The Society of Diagnostic Medical Sonographers, the written examination of The American Registry of Diagnostic Medical Sonographers, and many of the diagnostic ultrasound courses taught in North America is evidence of the agreement among many in this field that the subject is important. This inclusion should, in time, increase the understanding of the physical principles of diagnostic ultrasound by those in the field. A better understanding of the physical principles will reduce the occurrence of errors and misconceptions. A dozen regularly occurring errors and misconceptions are described in this section.

(1) "B-scan and real-time instruments each have advantages and disadvantages." The concern here is not with advantages and disadvantages, but with the incorrect distinction between B-scan and real-time or dynamic imaging instruments. The problem is that real-time instruments *are* B-scan instruments. It is true that A-mode and M-mode have always been real-time modes. But when one refers to real-time or dynamic imaging, it is a reference to dynamic two-dimensional cross-

sectional imaging, which is B-scan imaging. Thus, the distinction might better be made by saying "Static and dynamic instruments each have advantages and disadvantages." These, incidentally, are discussed in references 14–17.

(2) "An echo-free region on a display is a translucent or a transonic region." An echo-free region should be called echo-free or anechoic. Translucent means "shining through." Transonic, by analogy, implies that ultrasound passes through the region uninhibited. This is true only if attenuation is low. Absence of echoes does not guarantee this. It appears that, in general, reflection and scattering are minor contributors to attenuation (i.e., that absorption—conversion of sound to heat—is the major contributor). Absence of reflection or scattering does not reduce attenuation to zero, because the absorption component is still present. Therefore, to describe echo-free regions as being transonic is, in general, incorrect.

(3) "In the near zone, the beam diameter for a disc transducer is equal to the disc diameter" (Figure 11.1). This seems to have first occurred, without justification, in the acoustics textbook of Kinsler and Frey.[35] Zemanek[36] gives a more accurate picture of the ultrasound beam. Its characteristics in the near zone are complicated. It is desirable to provide a simplified, although approximate, picture of this behavior. Figure 11.1 is one such approach. However, a more accurate description is given in Figure 4.8, which indicates that the beam narrows to a minimum diameter at approximately the location of the transition from the near to the far zone. This picture approximates that portion of the sound that is greater than 4 percent of the spatial peak intensity occurring within the beam (Section 4.3). This particular value was chosen because it gives the simplest picture. The 6-dB beam diameter that is often used is narrower than that pictured in Figure 4.8. It includes that portion of the sound that is greater than 25 percent of the spatial peak intensity.

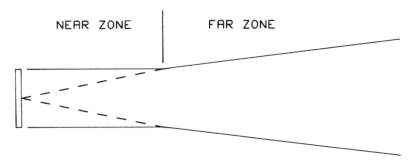

Figure 11.1. Traditional presentation of the beam for a flat disc transducer element. A more accurate view, using a 4 percent intensity beam diameter, is given in Figure 4.8.

It is important to realize that even for flat, unfocused transducer elements (Figures 4.8 and 11.1), there is some beam narrowing or "focusing." The beam diameter approximates the changing pulse diameter as an ultrasound pulse travels away from the transducer. With the 4 percent beam of Figure 4.8, this diameter reduces to approximately one-half of the transducer element diameter at the transition from near to far zone. The diameter then increases in the far zone.

(4) "Propagation speed increases with density." Propagation speed, in fact, decreases with increasing density if stiffness or bulk modulus remains constant. The dependence of the propagation speed, c, on density, ρ, and stiffness, M, is

$$c = \sqrt{\frac{M}{\rho}}$$

Since density is in the denominator, an increase in it produces a decrease in propagation speed. Density, ρ, is the concentration of mass; i.e., mass, m, divided by the volume, V, taken up by the mass (mass per unit volume). Stiffness, M, is a description of the resistance of a material to compression. It is equal to the applied pressure, p, divided by the fractional change in volume, ΔV_F, resulting from the pressure. The fractional volume change is the volume before the pressure was applied, V_1, minus the volume after the pressure was applied, V_2, all divided by the volume before the pressure was applied.

$$\rho = \frac{m}{V} \qquad M = \frac{p}{\Delta V_F} \qquad \Delta V_F = \frac{V_1 - V_2}{V_1}$$

If the material has a high stiffness, little change in volume will occur when pressure is applied. If it has low stiffness, a large change in volume will occur when pressure is applied.

It is generally true that media with higher densities also have higher stiffness, but this is not necessarily so. As an illustration, the propagation speed in brass is lower than that in aluminum even though the density of brass is approximately three times that of aluminum. In general, propagation speeds through gases are low, propagation speeds through liquids are higher, and propagation speeds through solids are the highest (Section 2.2). This *increasing* sequence is not caused by the increasing density (which produces a decreasing propagation speed) but by the increasing stiffness. This is because the stiffness differences are larger than the density differences.

(5) "The amplitude reflection, or pressure reflection, depends upon the impedance difference, $z_1 - z_2$." In this statement for perpendicular incidence (Figure 3.2), the subscripts are reversed and should appear as $z_2 - z_1$,

$$p_r \stackrel{..}{=} p_i \left[\frac{z_2 - z_1}{z_2 + z_1} \right] \qquad ARC \stackrel{..}{=} \frac{z_2 - z_1}{z_2 + z_1}$$

where p_r is reflected pressure, p_i is incident pressure, z_1 is medium one impedance, z_2 is medium two impedance, and ARC is the amplitude reflection coefficient. This error does not result in any change in the magnitude of the calculated reflection but will give a positive value when it should be negative and vice versa. A negative amplitude reflection indicates a reversal of polarity, so that the positive peaks are converted to negative and vice versa.

When calculating power or intensity reflection, the right-hand side of the equation is squared (Section 3.2),

$$I_r \overset{..}{=} I_i \left[\frac{z_2 - z_1}{z_2 + z_1} \right]^2 \qquad IRC \overset{..}{=} \left[\frac{z_2 - z_1}{z_2 + z_1} \right]^2$$

where I_r and I_i are reflected and incident intensity, respectively, and IRC is the intensity reflection coefficient. Since a negative number, when squared, becomes a positive number, the right-hand side of this equation is always positive. Therefore, it does not matter which way the subscripts are presented in the case of power or intensity reflection.

(6) "Reflections are produced by density differences." With perpendicular incidence, reflections are produced by impedance differences (changes in density or stiffness or both) (Section 3.2). The reflection amplitude is dependent on the impedances of the two media on either side of the boundary as shown in the equation in paragraph 5. Impedance is equal to density times propagation speed:

$$z = \rho c$$

For perpendicular incidence (Figure 3.2), a reflection is generated at a boundary if the impedances are different. A reflection may be generated when the densities are the same if the propagation speeds are different. On the other hand, no reflection may be generated even when the densities are different. This would be the case if the propagation speeds were different in the opposite direction by just the right amount to cancel the density differences (resulting in equal impedances). For example, if density is 1.01 on the left side and 1.00 on the right side while propagation speed is 1500 on the left and 1515 on the right, there is no reflection (for perpendicular incidence) even though the densities are different:

$$ARC \overset{..}{=} \frac{z_2 - z_1}{z_2 + z_1} = \frac{(1.00 \times 1515) - (1.01 \times 1500)}{(1.00 \times 1515) + (1.01 \times 1500)}$$

$$= \frac{1515 - 1515}{1515 + 1515} = \frac{0}{3030} = 0$$

(7) "Absence of reflection means that the media impedances are the same" or "If media impedances are the same there is no reflection." In the case of perpendicular incidence, as described in Section 3.2, these statements are true. In the case of oblique incidence, they gen-

erally are not (Section 3.3). Amplitude reflection for oblique incidence (Figure 3.3) is,

$$ARC = \frac{z_2 \cos \theta_i - z_1 \cos \theta_t}{z_2 \cos \theta_i + z_1 \cos \theta_t}$$

where θ_i and θ_t are incidence and transmission angles, respectively, and cos is cosine (Appendix C). With oblique incidence, it is possible for there to be no reflection even when media impedances are different. This would occur when the cosine factors in the equation are different in an opposite way, thus cancelling the effects of the impedance differences. For example, if $z_2 = 104$, $z_1 = 100$, $\cos \theta_i = 0.48$, and $\cos \theta_2 = 0.50$, then:

$$ARC = \frac{z_2 \cos \theta_i - z_1 \cos \theta_t}{z_2 \cos \theta_i + z_1 \cos \theta_t} = \frac{(104 \times 0.48) - (100 \times 0.50)}{(104 \times 0.48) + (100 \times 0.50)}$$

$$= \frac{50 - 50}{50 + 50} = \frac{0}{100} = 0$$

On the contrary, it is possible for there to be a reflection even when media impedances are equal. This would occur if the cosine terms were different, that is, when the propagation speeds of the two media are different.

(8) "Reflection amplitude decreases with increasing incidence angle." Whether this is true or not depends on the densities and propagation speeds involved. The relevant equation is given in paragraph 7. It is possible, with certain values of propagation speed and density, for the reflection amplitude to increase (Figure 11.2), decrease (Figure 11.3), or remain constant (Figure 11.4) as angle increases. The reflection amplitude may pass through a minimum and then increase (Figure 11.3) or start at zero (equal impedances) and increase (Figure 11.2).

(9) "Snell's law states that the angle of incidence equals the angle of reflection." These angles are indeed equal (Figure 3.3), but this is not Snell's law. Snell's law states the refraction relationship between the angles of incidence and transmission (Sections 3.3 and 11.2):

$$\sin \theta_t = \left[\frac{c_2}{c_1} \right] \sin \theta_i$$

(10) "The amplitude absorption coefficient is 3 dB/cm." Decibels are power or intensity ratio units (Appendix C). Therefore, when attenuation or absorption coefficients are expressed in dB, they are power or intensity, not amplitude, coefficients. The neper (Np) unit is used for expressing amplitude ratios.

*(11) "The **velocity** is 1540 m/s."* Velocity is the time rate of linear motion in a given direction. If a direction is not stated, then a speed, not velocity, has been specified.

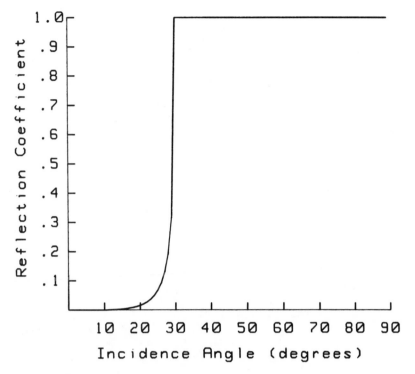

Figure 11.2. Intensity reflection coefficient as a function of incidence angle for impedances equal to 1 and 1 and propagation speeds equal to 1 and 2. There is no reflection for perpendicular incidence (incidence angle = 0) since the impedances are equal.

(12) *"This is a fluid-filled lung."* This use of the word, fluid, to mean liquid is common throughout medical imaging. A fluid is a material that flows or conforms to the outline of its container. Therefore, fluid means liquid or gas. Thus, lungs are *normally* fluid (air) filled.

Exercises

11.1.1. Propagation speed increases with increasing
    a. stiffness
    b. density
    c. absorption
    d. attenuation
    e. both a and b

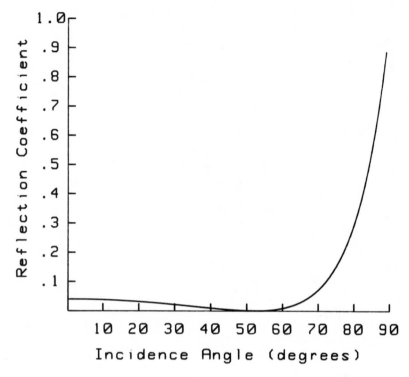

Figure 11.3. Intensity reflection coefficient as a function of incidence angle for impedances equal to 2 and 3 and propagation speeds equal to 2 and 1. At an incidence angle of about 50 degrees, there is no reflection, even though the impedances are not equal.

11.1.2. Reflections are produced by changes in
    a. stiffness
    b. density
    c. absorption
    d. attenuation
    e. both a and b

11.1.3. If no reflection occurs at a boundary, this always means that media impedances are equal in the case of
    a. perpendicular incidence
    b. oblique incidence
    c. refraction
    d. both a and b
    e. both b and c

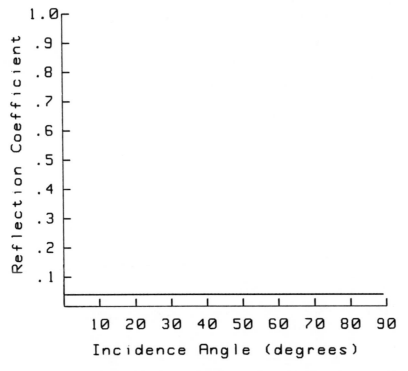

Figure 11.4. Intensity reflection coefficient as a function of incidence angle for impedances equal to 2 and 3 and propagation speeds equal to 1 and 1. The reflection coefficient is constant because the speeds are equal.

11.1.4. If the propagation speeds in two media are equal, Snell's law states that the incidence angle equals the
    a. reflection angle
    b. transmission angle
    c. Doppler angle
    d. both a and b
    e. both b and c

11.1.5. At a distance of one near-zone length from a disc transducer, the beam diameter is equal to the disc diameter divided by
    a. one
    b. two
    c. three
    d. π
    e. one-fourth

11.1.6. An echo-free region on a display is
   a. translucent
   b. transonic
   c. anechoic
   d. both a and b
   e. both b and c

11.1.7. Reflection coefficient _____ as incidence angle increases.
   a. increases
   b. stays constant
   c. decreases
   d. any of the above
   e. none of the above

11.1.8. A fluid is a _____ .
   a. gas
   b. liquid
   c. solid
   d. a or b
   e. b or c

11.1.9. Velocity is _____ .
   a. speed
   b. direction
   c. acceleration
   d. a and b
   e. all of the above

11.1.10. Decibels are _____ ratio units.
   a. amplitude
   b. power
   c. neper
   d. more than one of the above
   e. all of the above

11.1.11. Which of the following should be used in the numerator of the amplitude reflection equation?
   a. $(z_2 - z_1)^2$
   b. $(z_1 - z_2)^2$
   c. $(z_1 + z_2)^2$
   d. $z_1 + z_2$
   e. none of the above

11.1.12. Which of the following can be real-time? (More than one correct answer)
   a. A-mode
   b. B-mode
   c. B-scan
   d. M-mode
   e. Doppler

Many statements in this book are simplifications of the actual situation. They are used for simplicity and brevity. Clarification of some of these is given in this section. They are listed by relevant section numbers in the book.

2.2. Propagation speed is not quite independent of frequency. It increases slightly (about 1 m/s/MHz) with frequency in tissues. Since going from 2 to 10 MHz would only increase speed by about 8 m/s (0.5 percent), this fact can be ignored in imaging. Since propagation speed does increase slightly with frequency, impedance does also.

2.3 Frequency within pulses is not actually the same as that for continuous waves. A continuous wave may be described by a single frequency. Pulses have many frequencies present (see Figure 4.6). The shorter the pulse, the greater the bandwidth. The dominant frequency present in the pulse is close to or equal to the frequency for the unpulsed (cw) wave.

Pulse duration must be specified by some definition of where in time to stop. For example, a 10-dB pulse duration is the time during which the pulse intensity is one tenth or greater of the maximum occurring in the pulse.

2.4. Intensity *is* proportional to amplitude squared. The relationship is, where specific acoustic impedance is used (see 3.2 below).

$$\text{intensity} = \frac{(\text{pressure amplitude})^2}{2 \times \text{impedance}} \qquad I = \frac{A_p}{2 \times z}$$

$$= (\text{particle velocity amplitude})^2 \times \frac{\text{impedance}}{2} \qquad I = \frac{A_v \times z}{2}$$

2.5. Attenuation coefficients from laboratory measurements of in vitro tissue samples are given in Tables 2.4 and 2.5. This yields the approximate rule that tissue attenuation is 1 dB/cm/MHz of frequency. Although a true description of these laboratory data, this rule gives attenuation values larger than those encountered in medical imaging. There it appears that a value of 0.7 dB/cm/MHz may be more appropriate. Here the cm refers to sound travel path length. If imaging depth is used (half the path length, since the sound has to make a round trip), the figure, 1.4 dB/cm of depth per megahertz results. In a manner similar to half-intensity depth (Section 2.5) imaging depth can be calculated assuming 60 dB of compensation capability in the receiver. This yields:

$$\text{imaging depth (cm)} = \frac{43}{\text{frequency (MHz)}} \qquad D_I = \frac{43}{f}$$

Using this equation we expect to image to depths as follows:

2.25 MHz	19 cm
3.5	12
5.0	9
7.5	6
10.0	4

These appear to be reasonable values in practice. The reason for the discrepancy between the attenuation values from experimental measurements and from imaging practice is not clear.

3.2.   The impedance described in Section 2.2 is actually the characteristic acoustic impedance, which is *defined* as density times propagation speed. The impedance used in Section 3.2 is *not* the characteristic impedance, but rather the specific acoustic impedance, which is defined as pressure divided by particle velocity. The two impedances are equal for a plane (nondiverging or converging) wave is a nonattenuating medium.

3.3   The equation given as Snell's law is an approximation. The correct form is:

$$\text{sine of transmission angle (°)} = \frac{\text{sine of incidence angle (°)} \times \text{medium two propagation speed (mm/}\mu\text{s)}}{\text{medium one propagation speed (mm/}\mu\text{s)}} \qquad \sin \theta_t = \frac{c_2}{c_1} \times \sin \theta_i$$

For small incidence angles, the difference is not significant.

4.2.   The most general definition of a transducer is a device through which energy can flow from one medium or system to another. The energy conducted by these media or systems may be of the same or different forms. The latter case conforms to the transducer definition given in Section 4.2.

Bandwidth must be specified by some definition of where in the frequency range to stop. For example, a 6-dB bandwidth is the range of frequencies including those that have half or greater the amplitude of the strongest one (operating frequency).

4.3. The focal region must be specified by some definition of where in the beam to stop. For example, (1) a 6-dB focal region is the region in which the intensity at the beam center is 25 percent or greater of the spatial peak at the focus, or (2) the region in which the beam diameter is less than twice the minimum (at the focus).

The beam was presented in Figure 4.8 (a) for continuous-wave mode and used to describe pulses in the rest of the figure. The beam for pulses is not exactly the same as for continuous sound. One important reason for this is that the beam is a result of Huygens' principle, which states that each small portion of the surface of a transducer may be considered as a separate (omnidirectional) source. The beam is a result of combining the resulting sound emanating from all the small sources. For short pulses, this combination process is altered. Another reason why pulse beams are different is because pulses contain many frequencies. Since a beam depends on frequency, many beams are produced for a wide-bandwidth pulse. The combination of all of these results in the actual pulse beam produced. Since lateral resolution depends on beam diameter, which depends on pulse duration, axial and lateral resolutions are not independent.

4.4. Since ultrasound pulses used in imaging do not have constant amplitude (Figure 2.12), the overlapping and separation concept of resolution in Section 4.4 needs further discussion. How much can the pulses overlap and still be distinguished? This depends on the gray-scale resolution of the imaging system (Section 5.4). The better it is, the better the geometric (axial and lateral) resolution. This is because even with overlap, pulses can have a dip in their combined amplitude (Figure 11.5). If the gray-scale resolution of the system can sense this dip, the echoes can be resolved. Thus, gray-scale resolution and geometric resolution interact and are not independent. This also means that geometric resolutions are *related* to, not necessarily *equal* to, spatial pulse length and beam diameter.

5.1. Some authors consider a clock or timing circuit separately in a diagram such as Figure 5.2. The clock determines the pulse repetition frequency and causes the various components of the instrument to work together. In Figure 5.2 and in Sections 5.1 and 5.2, the clock is considered to be part of the pulser.

5.3. Since diagnostic ultrasound pulses do not have constant amplitude (Figure 2.12), when demodulated they do not have the blocked appearance shown in Figures 5.8 and 5.12 but rather appear as in Figure 11.5.

189

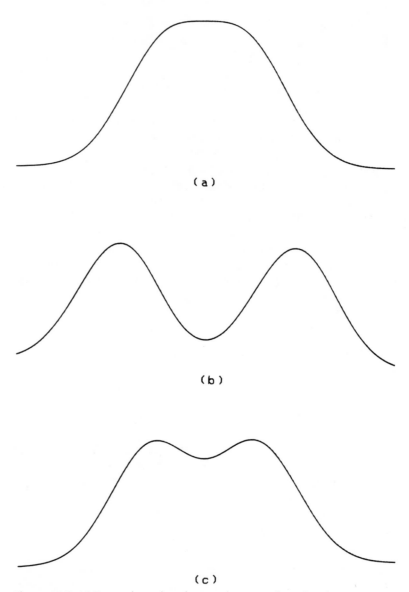

(a)

(b)

(c)

Figure 11.5. (a) Two echo pulses that overlap enough so that there is no amplitude dip between them. These cannot be distinguished by the instrument. They therefore will be presented as one and be unresolved. (b) Significantly less overlap (significantly greater reflector separation) than in (a) results in a large amplitude dip so that the echo pulses can be easily resolved even with poor gray-scale resolution. (c) With overlap intermediate between (a) and (b), a moderate amplitude dip occurs. This may or may not be detected (depending on the gray-scale resolution of the instrument). These echoes therefore (and the reflectors from which they originated) may or may not be resolved on the display.

7.2 The Doppler-shift equation should have the sum of propagation speed and reflector speed in the denominator. The use of propagation speed alone is an acceptable approximation because physiologic speeds are small compared with sound speed.

Chapter 12

Summary

By sending short pulses of ultrasound into the body and using reflected and scattered sound received from tissue interfaces and from within tissues to produce images of internal structures, ultrasound is used as a medical diagnostic tool. Ultrasound is a wave of traveling acoustic variables described by frequency, period, wavelength, propagation speed, amplitude, intensity, and attenuation.

Pulsed ultrasound is used in ultrasound imaging. It is described, additionally, by pulse repetition frequency and period, pulse duration, duty factor, and spatial pulse length. Pulses contain a range of frequencies described by bandwidth and Q. Diagnostic ultrasound commonly uses frequencies from 1 to 10 MHz, SPTA intensities from 0.01 to 200 mW/cm^2, pulse repetition frequencies from 0.5 to 4 kHz, duty factors from 0.001 to 0.003, and pulses of from 2 to 3 cycles. Soft-tissue propagation speed is 1.54 mm/μs and the attenuation coefficient is 1 dB/cm for each MHz of frequency.

For *perpendicular incidence* at boundaries, reflections are produced if media impedances (density $\times$ propagation speed) are different. For *oblique incidence,* refraction occurs if media propagation speeds are different. Scattering occurs at rough boundaries and within heterogeneous media. Scattering strength increases with increasing frequency. A Doppler shift is produced if a reflector or scatterer is moving. The distance to reflectors is determined by round-trip travel time.

Transducers convert electrical energy to ultrasound energy and vice versa by piezoelectricity. Axial resolution is equal to one half the spatial pulse length, which can be reduced by damping or increasing frequency (improving resolution). Lateral resolution is equal to beam diameter, which can be reduced by focusing (improving resolution). These resolutions (with focusing) are approximately 1 mm. Disc transducers produce sound beams with near and far zones. Focusing can only be accomplished in the near zone of the comparable unfocused transducer. Arrays can scan, steer, and shape beams repeatedly, permitting dynamic imaging. Dynamic imaging can also be accomplished with mechanically driven single-element transducers or mirrors.

Pulse-echo systems use the amplitude, direction, and arrival time of reflections to produce A-, B-, or M-mode displays. Imaging systems consist of pulser, transducer, receiver, memory, and display. Pulsers set the pulse repetition frequency, which determines maximum unambiguous imaging depth. Receivers amplify, compensate, demodulate, and compress echo voltage pulses. Scan converters store gray-scale image information and permit display on a television monitor. They are of two types—analog and digital. The number of bits per pixel in a digital memory determines the gray-scale resolution. Dynamic imaging instruments display a rapid sequence of static pictures. Doppler instruments use the Doppler shift of reflections to produce audible sound or images characteristic of motion. Pulsed Doppler instruments obtain range information. Spectral analysis provides a quantitative measure of Doppler information.

Display artifacts include resolution, texture, slice thickness, reverberation, curved and oblique reflectors, refraction, side and grating lobes, critical angle, multipath, mirror image, shadowing, enhancement, speed error, and range ambiguity.

Imaging performance is measured with test objects and TE phantoms. Acoustic output is measured with hydrophones. Beam profilers, test objects, and hydrophones measure transducer beam characteristics. Spectrum analyzers measure frequency content of ultrasound pulses.

There have been no independently confirmed significant bioeffects in mammalian tissues exposed to SPTA intensities below 100 mW/cm^2. Current data indicate that the benefits to patients of the prudent use of diagnostic ultrasound outweigh any potential risk.

Exercises

12.1. Increasing the frequency
   a. improves the resolution
   b. increases the half-intensity depth
   c. increases refraction
   d. both a and b
   e. both a and c

12.2. Increasing the pulse repetition frequency
  a. improves resolution
  b. increases maximum depth imaged unambiguously
  c. decreases maximum depth imaged unambiguously
  d. both a and b
  e. both a and c

12.3. Increasing the intensity produced by the transducer
  a. is accomplished by increasing the pulser voltage
  b. increases the sensitivity of the system
  c. increases the probablity of bioeffects
  d. all of the above
  e. none of the above

12.4. Increasing the spatial pulse length
  a. is accomplished by transducer damping
  b. is accompanied by decreased pulse duration
  c. improves axial resolution
  d. all of the above
  e. none of the above

12.5. Dynamic imaging is made possible by
  a. scan converters
  b. mechanically driven transducers
  c. gray-scale display
  d. arrays
  e. both b and d

12.6. The 100-mm test object measures
  a. resolution
  b. pulse duration
  c. SATA intensity
  d. wavelength
  e. all of the above

12.7. The following measure acoustic output:
  a. hydrophone
  b. scan converter
  c. 100-mm test object
  d. all of the above
  e. none of the above

12.8. Ultrasound bioeffects
  a. do not occur
  b. do not occur with diagnostic instruments
  c. are not confirmed below 100 mW/cm^2 SPTA
  d. both b and c
  e. none of the above

12.9. The diagnostic ultrasound frequency range is
   a. 1–10 mHz
   b. 1–10 kHz
   c. 1–10 MHz
   d. 3–15 kHz
   e. none of the above

12.10. Small transducers always produce smaller beam diameters. True or false?

12.11. No reflection occurs if media impedances are equal. True or false?

12.12. No refraction occurs if media impedances are equal. True or false?

12.13. Gray-scale display is made possible by
   a. array transducers
   b. cathode-ray storage tubes
   c. scan converters
   d. both b and c
   e. all of the above

12.14. Attenuation is corrected for by
   a. demodulation
   b. desegregation
   c. decompression
   d. compensation
   e. remuneration

12.15. Vertical deflections of the display spot are produced by reflections in
   a. the B mode
   b. the Doppler mode
   c. the M mode
   d. the à la mode
   e. none of the above

12.16. The Doppler effect for a scatterer moving toward the transducer causes scattered sound (compared with the incident sound) received by the transducer to have _____ .
   a. increased intensity
   b. decreased intensity
   c. increased impedance
   d. increased frequency
   e. decreased impedance

12.17. An ultrasound instrument that could represent 64 shades of gray would require an eight-bit memory. True or false?

12.18. Continuous-wave sound is used in _____ .
    a. all imaging instruments
    b. some imaging instruments
    c. all Doppler instruments
    d. some Doppler instruments
    e. none of the above

12.19. What is the transmitted intensity if the incident intensity is 1 and the impedances are 1.00 and 2.64?
    a. 0.2
    b. 0.4
    c. 0.6
    d. 0.8
    e. 1.0

12.20. Match the following (answers may be used more than once):
    a. A mode: _____, _____, _____   1. one-dimensional
    b. B scan: _____, _____, _____   2. two-dimensional
    c. M mode: _____, _____, _____   3. real-time
                                                  4. deflection
                                                 5. brightness
                                                 6. real-time or static

12.21. An advantage of continuous-wave-Doppler instruments is that they have _____ .
    a. no interaction with the pulse repetition frequency
    b. depth information
    c. bidirectional information
    d. amplitude information
    e. all of the above

12.22. An advantage of pulsed-Doppler instruments is that they have _____ .
    a. no interaction with the pulse repetition frequency
    b. depth information
    c. bidirectional information
    d. amplitude information
    e. all of the above

12.23. A digital memory with one bit per pixel would have a _____ display.
    a. bidirectional
    b. biscattering
    c. bistable
    d. bibonds
    e. bigeorge

12.24. If a transducer element, 19 mm in diameter, is focused to
produce a minimum beam diameter of 2 mm, the intensity
at the focus is approximately _____ times the intensity at
the transducer.
a. 2
b. 3
c. 19
d. 100
e. 500

12.25. The largest number that can be stored in a pixel of a seven-
bit digital memory is _____ .
a. 16
b. 32
c. 127
d. 255
e. 256

12.26. Digital calipers provide a measurement of distance between
_____ .
a. potentiometers
b. bits
c. optical encoders
d. pixels
e. all of the above

12.27. Which of the following produce(s) a sector-scan format?
a. rotating mechanical real-time transducer
b. oscillating mechanical real-time transducer
c. phased array
d. oscillating mirror
e. all of the above

12.28. A digital imaging instrument divides the cross-sectional
image into _____ .
a. frequencies
b. bits
c. pixels
d. binaries
e. wavelengths

12.29. Digital scan converters have better _____ than analog scan
converters.
a. spatial resolution
b. gray-scale resolution
c. sensitivity
d. reliability
e. efficiency

12.30. The binary number 10111 is equal to the decimal number
_____ .
a. 10
b. 16
c. 20
d. 23
e. 111

12.31. The axial resolution for a two-cycle pulse of 5 MHz in tissue
is _____ mm.
a. 0.1
b. 0.2
c. 0.3
d. 0.4
e. 0.5

12.32. The best lateral resolution for an unfocused 13 mm
transducer element is _____ mm.
a. 2.5
b. 4.5
c. 6.5
d. 815
e. 13

12.33. If the frequency of the element in Problem 12.32 is 3.5
MHz, the near-zone length is _____ cm.
a. 5
b. 10
c. 15
d. 20
e. 25

12.34. Can the element of Problem 12.33 be focused at 5 cm? Yes
or no?

12.35. If pulse repetition frequency is increased, the SPTA intensity
is _____ .
a. increased
b. unchanged
c. decreased
d. eliminated
e. none of the above

12.36. If the thickness of a transducer element is decreased, the
frequency is _____ .
a. increased
b. unchanged
c. decreased
d. intensified
e. none of the above

12.37. In problem 12.36, the near-zone length is _____.
   a. increased
   b. unchanged
   c. decreased
   d. intensified
   e. none of the above

12.38. With increased damping, which of the following is increased?
   a. bandwidth
   b. pulse duration
   c. spatial pulse length
   d. Q
   e. all of the above

12.39. As frequency is increased, which of the following are decreased?
   a. propagation speed
   b. half-intensity depth
   c. imaging depth
   d. more than one of the above
   e. none of the above

12.40. If a static image is produced by a 3 second scan, there will be approximately _____ scan lines in the image.
   a. 3
   b. 100
   c. 300
   d. 3000
   e. 30,000

12.41. If linear preprocessing is used and the echo dynamic range is 40 dB, a 20-dB echo will be assigned the number _____ in a six-bit memory.
   a. 0
   b. 16
   c. 32
   d. 48
   e. 64

12.42. If linear postprocessing is used, a stored 48 in a six-bit memory will produce _____ percent brightness on the display.
   a. 0
   b. 15
   c. 50
   d. 75
   e. 100

12.43. A five-bit memory can store which of the following numbers?
a. 64
b. 32
c. 31
d. 55
e. all of the above

12.44. Television monitors produce _____ frames per second.
a. 10
b. 24
c. 30
d. 60
e. none of the above

12.45. Duplex Doppler instruments include _____.
a. pulsed Doppler
b. cw Doppler
c. static imaging
d. dynamic imaging
e. more than one of the above

12.46. Match the following modes of display with the information that can be obtained:
a. A mode: _____, _____   1. reflector motion
b. M mode: _____, _____   2. reflector distance
c. static B scan: _____,   3. reflector shape
_____   4. reflector density
d. dynamic B scan:

_____, _____, _____

12.47. If the Doppler shifts from normal and stenotic carotid arteries are 4 kHz and 10 kHz, respectively, for which will there be a problem with a pulse repetition frequency of 7 kHz?
a. normal
b. stenotic
c. both
d. neither

12.48. Compensation (swept gain) makes up for the fact that reflections from deeper reflectors arrive at the transducer later. True or false?

12.49. Which of the following affects gray-scale resolution?
a. number of pixels
b. number of bits per pixel
c. pulse duration
d. frequency
e. focusing

12.50. Which of the following requires a phased array as a
receiving transducer?

a. dynamic range
b. dynamic imaging
c. dynamic focusing
d. dynamic personality
e. none of the above

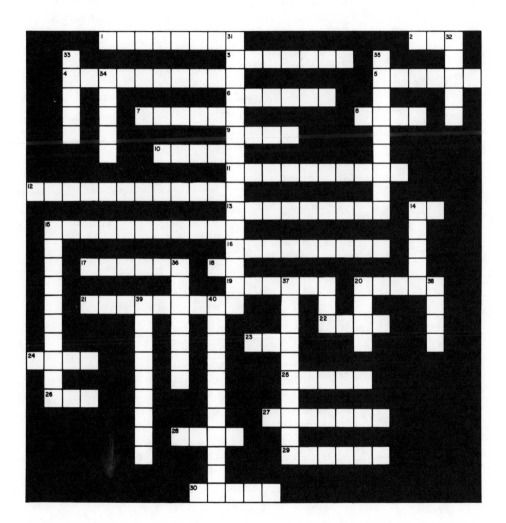

12.51. Across:

1. Referring to sound
2. Abbreviation for cosine
3. Not perpendicular to a boundary
4. Occurs at boundaries with perpendicular incidence
5. Material through which sound is passing
6. Pulsed Doppler requires _____ the receiver

7. The duty _____ is sound-on fraction
8. Beam diameter decreases in the _____ zone
9. Intensity is power divided by _____
10. Reflector motion produces a Doppler _____
11. Sound of frequency 20 kHz and higher
12. Parallel to sound direction
13. Maximum variation of an acoustic variable
14. Abbreviation for continuous wave
15. Attenuation _____ is given in decibels per centimeter
16. Power divided by area
17. Reciprocal of frequency
18. The range equation gives distance _____ a reflector
19. Perpendicular to a boundary
20. Displacement divided by time
21. Propagation speed depends on density and _____
22. _____ scale displays several values of spot brightness
23. Beam diameter increases in the _____ zone
24. Force times displacement
25. Axial resolution depends on spatial _____ length
26. Abbreviation for sine
27. Reflected frequency minus incident frequency equals
    _____ shift
28. A traveling variation
29. Capability for doing work
30. Complete variation of a wave variable

Down:
14. One hertz is one _____ per second.
15. The abbreviation cw stands for _____ wave
20. A line produced on a display is called a _____ line
31. (A message for you)
32. Traveling wave of acoustic variables
33. Transducer assembly containing more than one element
34. _____ length is the distance from a focused transducer
    to mimimum beam diameter
35. Density times propagation speed
36. Mass divided by volume
37. Another name for a hydrophone
38. Pulse duration divided by pulse repetition period is
    _____factor
39. Reciprocal of period
40. Ability of an imaging system to detect weak reflections

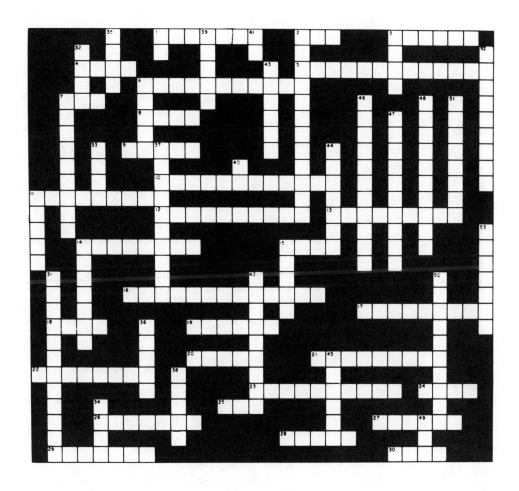

12.52. Across

1. Ratio of largest to smallest power that a system can handle is called _____ range.
2. At a distance of one near-field length from a disc transducer, beam diameter is approximately equal to disc diameter divided by _____.
3. Passing only reflections that arrive at a certain time after the transducer has produced a pulse is called _____.
4. Continuously displaying moving structures is called _____ time imaging.
5. Increasing small voltages to larger ones.
6. The speed with which a wave moves through a medium is called _____ speed.
7. The region of a sound beam where beam diameter increases with distance from the transducer is called the _____ zone.

8. Another word for a reflection.
9. Acoustics means having to do with _____.
10. If propagation speeds of two media are equal, Snell's law states that incidence angle equals _____ angle.
11. A device that stores a gray-scale image and allows it to be displayed on a television monitor is called a scan _____.
12. Conversion of sound to heat.
13. Power divided by area.
14. An echo-free region on a display is called _____.
15. The fraction of time that pulsed ultrasound is actually on is called _____ factor.
16. The AIUM statement on bioeffects says that there have been no _____ confirmed significant bioeffects below 100 mW/cm^2.
17. Density multiplied by sound propagation speed.
18. Displaying several values of spot brightness is carried out on a _____ scale.
19. If no reflection occurs at a boundary, this always means that media impedances are equal in the case of _____ incidence.
20. A few cycles of ultrasound may be called an ultrasound _____.
21. Maximum variation of an acoustic variable or voltage.
22. Reverberations are also called _____ reflections.
23. A device that converts energy from one form to another.
24. Prefix meaning 1000.
25. Abbreviation for megahertz.
26. _____ incidence is when the sound direction is not perpendicular to the boundary of the medium.
27. Capability of doing work.
28. Number of complete scans displayed per unit time in a real-time system is called the _____ rate.
29. Perpendicular to the direction of sound travel.
30. A unit for impedance.

Down
1. Abbreviation for decibel.
2. Sound _____ through a medium improves as attenuation decreases.

3. Ratio of output to input electric power for an amplifier.
6. A Greek prefix meaning pressure.
7. Number of cycles per unit time.
11. One hertz is one _____ per second.
14. An _____ array is made up of ring-shaped elements.
15. Half-intensity _____ decreases with increasing frequency.
31. Along the direction of sound travel (axial).
32. Focusing produces decreased beam _____.
33. A sound _____ is a traveling variation of acoustic variables.
34. Most two-dimensional imaging is done with B _____ displays.
35. To sweep a sound beam to produce an image.
36. Rate at which work is done; rate at which energy is transferred.
37. Sound of frequency greater than 20 kHz.
38. Concentrate the sound beam into a smaller area.
39. A transducer _____ is an assembly containing more than one transducer element.
40. Abbreviation for millimeter.
41. Abbreviation for continuous wave.
42. Frequency unit.
43. A _____ array is made up of rectangular elements in a line.
44. Propagation speed increases with decreasing _____.
45. Material through which a wave travels.
46. Decrease of amplitude and intensity as a wave travels through a medium.
47. Length of space over which a cycle occurs.
48. Change of sound direction on passing from one medium to another.
49. A cathode _____ tube is a common display device.
50. Diffusion or redirection of sound in several directions.
51. Speed, with direction of motion specified.
52. Perpendicular _____ occurs when sound direction is perpendicular to the boundary of the medium.
53. The _____ effect is a frequency change of reflected sound wave due to reflector motion.

Problem 12.52 from Kremkau FW: Crossword puzzle. Medical Ultrasound 4:38, 1980; reprinted by permission of John Wiley & Sons, Inc.

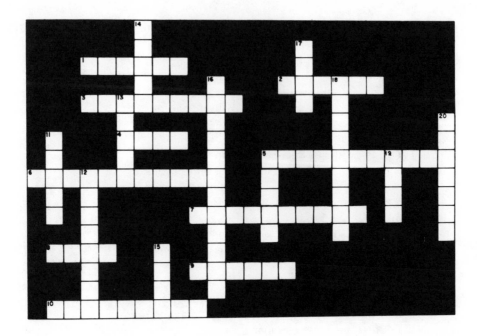

12.53. Identify the physical terms, the common measurement units for which are given.

Across
1. joule
2. microsecond
3. rayl
4. joule
5. decibel
6. kelvin
7. millimeter
8. gram
9. milliliter
10. hertz

Down
5. radian
11. meter/second
12. newton/meter^2
13. watt
14. newton
15. decibel
16. meter/second^2
17. centimeter^2
18. watt/centimeter^2
19. second
20. gram/milliliter

Problem 12.53 from Kremkau FW: Ultrapuzzles. Reflections 6:85, 1980; reprinted by permission of the American Institute of Ultrasound in Medicine.

12.54. In the following review, blanks need to be filled in. In the figure, begin at the upper left and draw a line to one letter at a time in any direction (horizontal, vertical, or diagonal) to spell out the words for the blanks. Do not cross over your line. Use each letter only once. The words should be found in the same order as they are needed for the blanks.

Ultrasound is a _____ of traveling _____ variables. Pulsed ultrasound is commonly used in ultrasound imaging. Pulses contain a range of _____. Soft-tissue _____ _____ is 1.54 mm/μs and the _____ coefficient is 1 dB/cm for each _____ of frequency. _____ occurs at rough boundaries and within heterogeneous media. _____ convert electrical energy to ultrasound energy and vice versa. Imaging systems consist of pulser, transducer, receiver, _____, and _____. Dynamic-imaging instruments display a rapid _____ of static pictures.

START

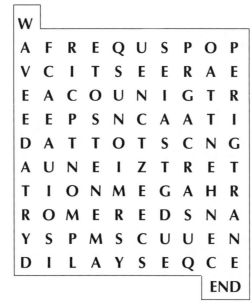

12.55. This textbook is
   a. enjoyable
   b. profitable
   c. relevant
   d. well done
   e. complete
   f. accurate
   g. concise
   h. stimulating
   i. simple
   j. clear
   k. error-freee
   m. omission-free
   o. helpful
   p. great
   q. perfect
   r. all of the above

Glossary

The terms defined here appear in **boldface** at first appearance in this book. Other definitions are found in references 37–39.

Absorption. Conversion of sound to heat.

Acceleration. Change in velocity divided by time over which the change occurs.

Acoustic. Having to do with sound.

Acoustic propagation properties. Characteristics of a medium that affect the propagation of sound through it.

Acoustic variables. Pressure, density, temperature, and particle motion—things that are functions of space and time in a sound wave.

A mode. Mode of operation in which the display records a vertical spot deflection for each pulse delivered from the receiver.

Amplification. Increasing small voltages to larger ones.

Amplifier. A device that accomplishes amplification.

Amplitude. Maximum variation of an acoustic variable or voltage.

Analog. Related to a procedure or system in which data are represented by continuously variable physical quantities (e.g., electric charge).

Annular array. Array made up of ring-shaped elements arranged concentrically.

Array. Transducer array.

Attenuation. Decrease in amplitude and intensity as a wave travels through a medium.

Attenuation coefficient. Attenuation per unit length of wave travel.

Axial. In the direction of the transducer axis (sound-travel direction).

Axial resolution. Minimum reflector separation along the sound path required for separate reflections to be produced.

Backscatter. Sound scattered back in the direction from which it originally came.

Bandwidth. Range of frequencies contained in an ultrasound pulse.

Beam area. Cross-sectional area of a sound beam.

Beam profiler. A device that plots three-dimensional reflection amplitude information.

Beam-uniformity ratio. Ratio of the spatial-peak to spatial-average intensity.

Bidirectional. Indicating Doppler instruments capable of distinguishing between positive and negative Doppler shifts (forward and reverse flow).

Bistable. Having two possible states (e.g., on or off; white or black).

Bistable display. Display in which all recorded spots have the same brightness.

Bit. Binary digit.

B mode. Mode of operation in which the display records a spot brightening for each echo pulse delivered from the receiver.

B scan. A brightness image that represents a cross section of the object through the scanning plane.

Cathode-ray tube. A display device that produces an image by scanning an electron beam over a phosphor-coated screen.

Cavitation (acoustic). Production and behavior of bubbles in sound.

Compensation. Equalizing received reflection amplitude differences caused by reflector depth.

Compressibility. Ability of a material to be reduced to a smaller volume under external pressure.

Compression. Decreasing differences between small and large amplitudes.

Continuous mode. Continuous-wave mode.

Continuous wave. A wave in which cycles repeat indefinitely, not pulsed.

Continuous-wave mode. Mode of operation in which continuous-wave sound is used.

cos. Abbreviation for cosine.

Cosine. The cosine of angle A in Figure C.1 is the length of side b divided by the length of side c.

Coupling medium. Oil or gel used to provide a good sound path between the transducer and the skin.

cw. Abbreviation for continuous wave.

Cycle. Complete variation of an acoustic variable.

Damping. Material placed behind the rear face of a transducer element to reduce pulse duration; also, the process of pulse duration reduction.

dB Abbreviation for decibel.

Dead zone. Distance close to the transducer in which imaging cannot be performed.

Decibel. Unit of power or intensity ratio; the number of decibels is 10 times the logarithm (to the base 10) of the power or intensity ratio.

Demodulation. Converting voltage pulses from one form to another.

Density. Mass divided by volume.

Digital. Related to a procedure or system in which data are represented by discrete units (numerical digits).

Disc. Thin flat circular object.

Displacement. Distance that an object has moved.

Doppler effect. Frequency change of reflected sound wave as a result of reflector motion relative to transducer.

Doppler shift. Reflected frequency minus incident frequency.

Duty factor. Fraction of time that pulsed ultrasound is actually on.

Dynamic focusing. Continuously variable received focus that follows the changing position of the transmitted pulse.

Dynamic imaging. Rapid-frame-sequence imaging.

Dynamic range. Ratio (in decibels) of largest power to smallest power that a system can handle or of the largest to the smallest intensity of a group of echoes.

Echo. Reflection.

Effective reflecting area. The area of a reflector from which sound is received by a transducer.

Electrical resistor. A device that limits the electric current for a given voltage.

Electric current. The rate of flow of electrons in an electrical conductor.

Electric pulse. A brief excursion of electric voltage from its normal value.

Electric resistance. The characteristic of electrical components that limits the electric current for a given voltage.

Electric voltage. Electric potential or potential difference expressed in volts.

Electricity. A form of energy associated with the displacement or flow of electrons.

Energy. Capability of doing work.

Enhancement. Increase in reflection amplitude from reflectors that lie behind a weakly attenuating structure.

Far zone. The region of a sound beam in which the beam diameter increases as the distance from the transducer increases.

Focal length. Distance from focused transducer to center of focal region or to the location of the spatial peak intensity.

Focal region. Region of minimum beam diameter and area.

Focus. To concentrate the sound beam into a smaller beam area than would exist otherwise.

Force. That which changes the state of rest or motion of an object.

Fractional bandwidth. Bandwidth divided by operating frequency.

Frame. Display image produced by one complete scan of the sound beam.

Frame rate. Number of frames displayed per unit time.

Frequency. Number of cycles per unit time.

Gain. Ratio of output to input electrical power.

Generator gate. The electronic portion of a pulsed Doppler system that converts the continuous voltage of the voltage generator to a pulsed voltage.

Grating lobes. Additional minor beams of sound traveling out in directions different from the primary beam. These result from the multielement structure of transducer arrays.

Gray scale. Continuous range of brightnesses between white and black.

Gray-scale display. Display in which several values of spot brightness may be displayed.

Gray-scale resolution. Ability of a gray-scale display to distinguish between echoes of slightly different amplitude or intensity.

Half-intensity depth. Depth in tissue at which intensity is reduced to one-half what it was at the surface.

Heat. Energy resulting from thermal molecular motion.

Hertz. Unit of frequency, one cycle per second; unit of pulse repetition frequency, one pulse per second.

Hydrophone. A small transducer element mounted on the end of a narrow tube.

Hz. Abbreviation for hertz.

Incidence angle. Angle between incident sound direction and line perpendicular to boundary of the medium.

Impedance. Density multiplied by sound propagation speed.

Intensity. Power divided by area.

Intensity reflection coefficient. Reflected intensity divided by incident intensity.

Intensity transmission coefficient. Transmitted intensity divided by incident intensity.

Internal focus. A focus produced by a curved transducer element.

kHz. Abbreviation for kilohertz.

Kilohertz. One thousand hertz.

Lateral. Perpendicular to the direction of sound travel.

Lateral resolution. Minimum reflector separation perpendicular to the sound path required for separate reflections to be produced.

Linear array. Array made up of rectangular elements in a line.

Linear phased array. Linear array operated by applying voltage pulses to all elements, but with small time differences.

Linear switched array. Linear array operated by applying voltage pulses to groups of elements sequentially.

log. Abbreviation for logarithm.

Logarithm. The logarithm of a number is equal to the number of tens that must be multiplied together to result in that number.

Longitudinal wave. Wave in which the particle motion is parallel to the direction of wave travel.

Mass. Measure of an object's resistance to acceleration.

Matching layer. Material placed in front of the front face of a transducer element to reduce the reflection at the transducer surface.

Medium. Material through which a wave travels.

Megahertz. One million hertz.

MHz. Abbreviation for megahertz.

M mode. Mode of operation in which the display presents a spot brightening for each pulse delivered from the receiver, producing a two-dimensional recording of reflector position (motion) versus time.

Multipath. Paths to and from a reflector are not the same.

Multiple reflection. Several reflections produced by a pulse encountering a pair of reflectors.

Near zone. The region of a sound beam in which the beam diameter decreases as the distance from the transducer increases.

Oblique incidence. Sound direction is not perpendicular to media boundary.

Operating frequency. Preferred frequency of operation of a transducer.

Particle. Small portion of a medium.

Particle motion. Displacement, speed, velocity, and acceleration of a particle.

Period. Time per cycle.

Perpendicular. Geometrically related by 90 degrees.

Perpendicular incidence. Sound direction is perpendicular to media boundary.

Piezoelectricity. Conversion of pressure to electric voltage.

Pixel. Picture element. The unit into which imaging information is divided for storage and display in a digital instrument.

Power. Rate at which work is done; rate at which energy is transferred.

Preamplifier. A device that performs some amplification on electric voltages close to the transducer before they travel along the cable to the instrument.

Pressure. Force divided by area.

Probe. Transducer assembly.

Propagation. Progression or travel.

Propagation speed. Speed with which a wave moves through a medium.

Pulse. A brief excursion of a quantity from its normal value; a few cycles.

Pulsed mode. Mode of operation in which pulsed ultrasound is used.

Pulsed ultrasound. Ultrasound produced in pulse form by applying electrical pulses to the transducer.

Pulse duration. Time from beginning to end of a pulse.

Pulse-echo diagnostic ultrasound. Ultrasound imaging in which pulses are reflected and used to produce a display.

Pulse repetition frequency. Number of pulses per unit time. Sometimes called pulse repetition rate.

Pulse repetition period. Time from the beginning of one pulse to the beginning of the next.

Quality factor. Operating frequency divided by bandwidth.

Range equation. Relationship between round-trip pulse travel time and distance to a reflector.

Rayl. Unit of impedance.

Real time. Imaging with a real-time display.

Real-time display. A display that continuously images moving structures.

Receiver gate. A device that allows only echoes from a selected depth (arrival time) to pass.

Reflection. Portion of sound returned from a boundary of a medium.

Reflection angle. Angle between reflected sound direction and line perpendicular to boundary of a medium.

Reflector. Medium boundary that produces a reflection; reflecting surface.

Refraction. Change of sound direction on passing from one medium to another.

Registration. Positioning of reflectors in the display.

Rejection. Eliminating smaller-amplitude voltage pulses.

Resonance frequency. Operating frequency.

Reverberation. Multiple reflections.

Scanning. Sweeping a sound beam to produce an image.

Scan converter. A device that stores imaging information in one scanning format and reads it out for display in another.

Scan line. A line produced on a display by moving a spot (produced by an electron beam) across the display face at constant speed.

Scatterer. An object that scatters sound because of its small size or its surface roughness.

Scattering. Diffusion or redirection of sound in several directions on encountering a particle suspension or a rough surface.

Sensitivity. Ability of an imaging system to detect weak reflections.

Shadowing. Reduction in reflection amplitude from reflectors that lie behind a strongly reflecting or attenuating structure.

Side lobes. Minor beams of sound traveling out in directions different from the primary beam.

sin. Abbreviation for sine.

Sine. The sine of angle A in Figure A3.1 is the length of side a divided by the length of side c.

Snell's law. An equation that relates incidence and transmission angles of refraction.

Sound. Traveling wave of acoustic variables.

Sound beam. The region of a medium that contains virtually all the sound produced by a transducer.

Spatial pulse length. Length of space over which a pulse occurs.

Speckle. The granular appearance of images caused by the interference of echoes from the distribution of scatterers in tissue.

Specular reflection. Reflection from a smooth boundary.

Speed. Displacement divided by time over which displacement occurs.

Static imaging. Single-frame imaging.

Stiffness. Property of a medium: applied pressure divided by fractional volume change produced by the pressure.

Strength. Nonspecific term referring to amplitude or intensity.

Temperature. Condition of a body that determines transfer of heat to or from other bodies.

Transducer. Device that converts energy from one form to another.

Transducer array. Transducer assembly containing more than one transducer element.

Transducer assembly. Transducer element and damping and matching materials assembled in a case.

Transducer element. Piece of piezoelectric material in a transducer assembly.

Transmission angle. Angle between transmitted sound direction and line perpendicular to boundary of a medium.

Ultrasound. Sound of frequency greater than 20 kHz.

Ultrasound transducer. Device that converts electric energy to ultrasound energy and vice versa.

Variable focusing. Transmit focus with various focal lengths.

Velocity. Speed with direction of motion specified.

Voltage pulse. Brief excursion of voltage from its normal value.

Wave. Traveling variation of wave variables.

Wavelength. Length of space over which a cycle occurs.

Wave variables. Things that are functions of space and time in a wave.

Work. Force multiplied by displacement.

Answers to Exercises in Text

Chapter 1

1.2.1. pulses, ultrasound, reflections, image
1.2.2. ultrasound, tissues
1.2.3. acoustic, diagnostic
1.2.4. bioeffects
1.2.5. a. 4; b. 3; c. 6; d. 1; e. 5; f. 2
1.2.6. a. 3; b. 1; c. 2

Chapter 2

2.2.1. wave variables
2.2.2. acoustic variables
2.2.3. 20,000
2.2.4. pressure, density, temperature, particle motion
2.2.5. c, d, e
2.2.6. a, e
2.2.7. cycles
2.2.8. hertz, Hz
2.2.9. time
2.2.10. reciprocal
2.2.11. space
2.2.12. wave
2.2.13. propagation speed, frequency
2.2.14. density, stiffness

2.2.15.	e
2.2.16.	1540, 1.54
2.2.17.	e
2.2.18.	a, c, b
2.2.19.	1.54
2.2.20.	decreases
2.2.21.	10
2.2.22.	higher
2.2.23.	d
2.2.24.	b
2.2.25.	higher
2.2.26.	mechanical longitudinal
2.2.27.	doubled
2.2.28.	1
2.2.29.	unchanged
2.2.30.	energy
2.2.31.	e
2.2.32.	false
2.2.33.	true
2.2.34.	1,540,000 (propagation speed is 1540 m/s)
2.2.35.	true
2.2.36.	true
2.2.37.	density, propagation speed
2.3.1.	continuous wave
2.3.2.	pulses
2.3.3.	pulses
2.3.4.	pulses
2.3.5.	period
2.3.6.	reciprocal
2.3.7.	time
2.3.8.	length, space
2.3.9.	Duty factor
2.3.10.	period
2.3.11.	wavelength
2.3.12.	1(100%)
2.3.13.	6
2.3.14.	2
2.3.15.	1.3 (period is 0.33 μs, soft tissue is irrelevant)
2.3.16.	1
2.3.17.	0.0013
2.3.18.	d
2.3.19.	c
2.3.20.	b
2.4.1.	variation
2.4.2.	power, area

2.4.3. W/cm^2
2.4.4. amplitude
2.4.5. doubled
2.4.6. halved
2.4.7. unchanged
2.4.8. quadrupled
2.4.9. 5
2.4.10. peak, average
2.4.11. average, peak
2.4.12. b
2.4.13. a. 3; b. 1; c. 3
2.4.14. 2
2.4.15. 3, 4

2.5.1. amplitude, intensity
2.5.2. absorption, reflection, scattering
2.5.3. length
2.5.4. dB, dB/cm
2.5.5. 1
2.5.6. 3 dB/cm
2.5.7. increases
2.5.8. doubled, doubled, quadrupled
2.5.9. unchanged
2.5.10. sound, heat
2.5.11. No (absorption is one part of attenuation)
2.5.12. Higher
2.5.13. 50, 1.5, 50, 1
2.5.14. 0.6
2.5.15. 5
2.5.16. attenuation coefficient
2.5.17. decreases
2.5.18. 0.32 (intensity ratio is 0.16), 1.5
2.5.19. 0.00000002
2.5.20. d

2.6.1. a
2.6.2. e
2.6.3. a. 4; b. 1; c. 3; d. 5; e. 2
2.6.4. a. 2; b. 3; c. 4; d.1
2.6.5. a. 3; b. 4; c. 1; d. 2; e. 5; f. 7; g. 6
2.6.6. a. 3; b. 4; c. 1; d. 2; e. 1; f. 3; g. 1; h. 5; i. 8; j. 7;
k. 6; l. 9; m. 4
2.6.7. a. 1; b. 2, 3; c. 3; d. 1; e. 2
2.6.8. a. 1.54; b. 0.77; c. 3.1; d. 0.5; e. 2; f. 1; g. 0.002; h. 2;
i. 2; j. 1.5; k. 6; l. 0.25; m. 0.25; n. 1; o. 125; p. 500;
q. 1,630,000

2.6.9. c

2.6.10. a

2.6.11. increased

Chapter 3

3.2.1. impedances

3.2.2. impedances, intensity

3.2.3. impedances

3.2.4. 0.0008, 1.9992

3.2.5. 0.0002, 1.9998

3.2.6. 0.0008, 1.9992

3.2.7. 0.01, 1 (incident intensity not needed)

3.2.8. 0.99, 99

3.2.9. 20 (intensity ratio 0.01, use Table C.2)

3.2.10. 0.01

3.2.11. 0 (impedances are equal)

3.2.12. 5, 0

3.2.13. True

3.2.14. False, in general (true only if propagation speeds are also equal)

3.2.15. False, in general (true only if densities are also equal)

3.2.16. False

3.2.17. 0.9990

3.2.18. air, reflection

3.2.19. 0.01

3.2.20. 0.43

3.2.21. d

3.3.1. direction

3.3.2. larger than, equal to

3.3.3. smaller than, equal to

3.3.4. equal to, equal to

3.3.5. 30, 21

3.3.6. 30, 30

3.3.7. 30, 39

3.3.8. 0.04 (incidence angle and intensity are not needed; the propagation speeds are equal, so that the calculation is the same as with perpendicular incidence)

3.3.9. 0.2 (no refraction; calculate as with perpendicular incidence)

3.3.10. perpendicular incidence, media propagation speeds are equal

3.3.11. media propagation speeds are equal (no refraction)

3.3.12. density, propagation speed

3.3.13. 32

3.3.14. 1.7

222

3.4.1. scattering
3.4.2. True
3.4.3. False
3.4.4. a
3.4.5. True
3.4.6. c

3.5.1. pulses, echoes, display
3.5.2. propagation speed, time
3.5.3. 4
3.5.4. 7
3.5.5. 7.7
3.5.6. 1

3.6.1. propagation speeds, equal
3.6.2. d
3.6.3. e
3.6.4. d
3.6.5. 0.04
3.6.6. impedances
3.6.7. densities or impedances, propagation speeds
3.6.8. 18
3.6.9. 23
3.6.10. False

Chapter 4

4.2.1. energy
4.2.2. electric, ultrasound
4.2.3. piezoelectricity
4.2.4. discs
4.2.5. thickness
4.2.6. element, assembly
4.2.7. element, assembly
4.2.8. continuous-wave
4.2.9. pulses
4.2.10. decreases
4.2.11. cycles, axial resolution, bandwidth, quality factor
4.2.12. efficiency, sensitivity
4.2.13. two, three
4.2.14. 0.2
4.2.15. 15
4.2.16. reflection
4.2.17. air
4.2.18. e
4.2.19. False

4.2.20. frequencies
4.2.21. c
4.2.22. a. 3; b. 0.33; c. 2.5; d. 3.5; e. 3

4.3.1. 4
4.3.2. near, far
4.3.3. near-zone
4.3.4. frequency or wavelength, diameter, distance
4.3.5. transducer diameter, wavelength
4.3.6. transducer diameter, frequency
4.3.7. one-half
4.3.8. two
4.3.9. decreases
4.3.10. increases
4.3.11. 30
4.3.12. 4.5, 3, 6, 12
4.3.13. 60
4.3.14. 3, 6, 9
4.3.15. longer, smaller
4.3.16. 120
4.3.17. 9, 6, 9, 12
4.3.18. longer, smaller
4.3.19. quadruples
4.3.20. doubles
4.3.21. doubled
4.3.22. e
4.3.23. False
4.3.24. Focal length

4.4.1. sound travel, reflections
4.4.2. spatial pulse length
4.4.3. True
4.4.4. 1.5
4.4.5. 1
4.4.6. 2.3, 0.2
4.4.7. halved
4.4.8. doubled
4.4.9. False
4.4.10. False
4.4.11. 1
4.4.12. 10 (less than 10 MHz in many applications)
4.4.13. wavelength, spatial pulse length
4.4.14. attenuation
4.4.15. separation, reflections
4.4.16. beam diameter or width

4.4.17. c, d, f
4.4.18. True
4.4.19. True
4.4.20. False (only true near the transducer)
4.4.21. b, c, e, f

4.5.1. a. 4; b. 3; c. 2; d. 1
4.5.2. a, d
4.5.3. a. 5; b. 0.3; c. 141; d. 6.5; e. 13
4.5.4. c
4.5.5. one-half, near-zone
4.5.6. focal
4.5.7. 6.5 (frequency not needed)
4.5.8. 0.7 (diameter not needed)
4.5.9. True
4.5.10. False
4.5.11. focal
4.5.12. True
4.5.13. False
4.5.14. a. 1, 2, 3; b. 2; c. 2; d. 1
4.5.15. a
4.5.16. e
4.5.17. a
4.5.18. b, c, d
4.5.19. True
4.5.20. Resolution, half-intensity depth
4.5.21. 1, 10
4.5.22. 1, 1.5

Chapter 5

5.1.1. pulser, transducer, receiver, memory, display
5.1.2. a. 4; b. 1; c. 2; d. 5; e. 3
5.1.3. a. 2; b. 2; c. 2, 3; d. 3; e. 1; f. 1; g. 2; h. 1, 2; i. 2, 3; j. 2, 3; k. 1, 2; l. 1, 2; m. 2, 3; n. 2, 3; o. 2, 3; p. 2, 3

5.2.1. pulse
5.2.2. amplitude, intensity
5.2.3. a. 3; b. 5; c. 1; d. 2; e. 4

5.3.1. amplification, compensation, demodulation, compression, rejection
5.3.2. a. 2; b. 5; c. 1; d. 3; e. 4
5.3.3. 10, 100, 20
5.3.4. 1
5.3.5. 10
5.3.6. b, e

5.3.7. depth, distance
5.3.8. times
5.3.9. dynamic, display
5.3.10. 2.0
5.3.11. pulses
5.3.12. False
5.3.13. a

5.4.1. a. 5; b. 3; c. 2; d. 1; e. 4
5.4.2. a
5.4.3. c
5.4.4. a. 5; b. 3; c. 2; d. 6; e. 1; f. 4
5.4.5. e
5.4.6. a. 4; b. 5; c. 6; d. 7; e. 8
5.4.7. d
5.4.8. d
5.4.9. e
5.4.10. a

5.5.1. A, B, M, B
5.5.2. a. 2, 7; b. 3, 7; c. 3, 4, 7; d. 1, 3, 5, 6
5.5.3. cathode-ray
5.5.4. deflection
5.5.5. time, distance or depth
5.5.6. True
5.5.7. M
5.5.8. time, propagation speed
5.5.9. scanning
5.5.10. gray-scale
5.5.11. scan converter
5.5.12. c
5.5.13. d
5.5.14. 33
5.5.15. 63

5.6.1. a
5.6.2. b
5.6.3. d
5.6.4. c
5.6.5. d
5.6.6. b, f, d, c, e, a
5.6.7. b
5.6.8. b
5.6.9. d
5.6.10. e
5.6.11. b

5.6.12. reflections or echoes
5.6.13. reflection or pulse-echo
5.6.14. pulse-echo
5.6.15. strength, direction, time
5.6.16. a
5.6.17. display, voltages or pulses
5.6.18. receiver
5.6.19. pulser
5.6.20. receiver
5.6.21. a
5.6.22. f
5.6.23. b
5.6.24. e
5.6.25. c
5.6.26. d
5.6.27. c
5.6.28. b
5.6.29. a
5.6.30. False

Chapter 6

6.2.1. element
6.2.2. linear, annular
6.2.3. switched, phased
6.2.4. a. 1; b. 2, 3; c. 2, 3; d. 3, 1, 2; e. 1, 2, 3
6.2.5. one
6.2.6. two
6.2.7. oscillating mirror
6.2.8. a. 1; b. 2; c. 2
6.2.9. b
6.2.10. a
6.2.11. c

6.3.1. a. 1; b. 2; c. 2; d. 2; e. 1; f. 2
6.3.2. 40
6.3.3. 1200
6.3.4. 4, 4
6.3.5. 0.4, 0.4

6.4.1. A, M
6.4.2. B
6.4.3. mechanical, electronic
6.4.4. frame
6.4.5. pulsed
6.4.6. lines, frame
6.4.7. False (latter portion)

7.2.1. frequency, motion
7.2.2. higher
7.2.3. lower
7.2.4. equal to
7.2.5. motion
7.2.6. 0.02, 1.02
7.2.7. 0.026
7.2.8. -0.026
7.2.9. reflected, incident
7.2.10. cosine
7.2.11. 0.01, 1.01 (the Doppler shift is cut in half)
7.2.12. 0, 1.00 (no Doppler shift at 90 degrees)

7.3.1. False
7.3.2. direction, bidirectional
7.3.3. False
7.3.4. voltage generator, source transducer, receiving transducer, receiver, loudspeaker
7.3.5. False (common Doppler shifts *are* in the audible frequency range)
7.3.6. False
7.3.7. False
7.3.8. False (it represents motion or flow under the surface scanned)

7.4.1. gates, transducers
7.4.2. continuous, pulsed
7.4.3. depths, arrival time
7.4.4. False
7.4.5. profile
7.4.6. True
7.4.7. a
7.4.8. gates

7.5.1. amplitude, frequency
7.5.2. frequency, time
7.5.3. gray, color
7.5.4. bandwidth, flow velocities
7.5.5. True

7.6.1. Doppler shift
7.6.2. False
7.6.3. one, two
7.6.4. frequencies
7.6.5. False
7.6.6. motion
7.6.7. gate

7.6.8.   display
7.6.9.   gate, voltage generator
7.6.10. depth
7.6.11. True
7.6.12. False
7.6.13. True
7.6.14. 2.6
7.6.15. True
7.6.16. cw

Chapter 8

8.2.1.   5.1
8.2.2.   77
8.2.3.   c
8.2.4.   False
8.2.5.   e
8.2.6.   a
8.2.7.   False. This is the display of the interference pattern of scattered sound from the distribution of scatterers in the tissue.
8.2.8.   slice thickness
8.2.9.   c, d, e, f
8.2.10. True

8.3.1.   a. 1; b. 2, 3; c. 3; d. 3; e. 2, 3; f. 4, 5; g. 4, 5; h. 4, i. 2, 6
8.3.2.   separation
8.3.3.   weaker
8.3.4.   b
8.3.5.   d
8.3.6.   True
8.3.7.   b
8.3.8.   192
8.3.9.   3.8
8.3.10. no (200 × 25 × 20 = 100,000: greater than 77,000)

Chapter 9

9.2.1.   rods, water, alcohol
9.2.2.   a. 1; b. 2; c. 3; d. 6; e. 4; f. 3; g. 7; h. 7
9.2.3.   a. 5; b. 5; c. 4; d. 3; e. 2; f. 1; g. 1; h. 1
9.2.4.   True
9.2.5.   True
9.2.6.   1
9.2.7.   distance

9.2.8. distances or depths
9.2.9. tissues
9.2.10. False

9.3.1. d
9.3.2. False
9.3.3. b
9.3.4. d

9.4.1. b, c, d, e
9.4.2. True
9.4.3. transducer
9.4.4. True
9.4.5. b
9.4.6. a. 2, 12 or 1, 9; b. 3, 12; c. 3, 8; d. 4 or 2, 9; e. 1, 7;
f. 5, 10; g. 6, 11

9.5.1. a. 2; b. 1, 2; c. 2, 3
9.5.2. a. 2; b. 3; c. 1

Chapter 10

10.4.1. False
10.4.2. False
10.4.3. b
10.4.4. No
10.4.5. Yes
10.4.6. a
10.4.7. a
10.4.8. b
10.4.9. e
10.4.10. False
10.4.11. d

Chapter 11

11.1.1. a
11.1.2. e
11.1.3. a
11.1.4. b
11.1.5. b
11.1.6. c
11.1.7. d
11.1.8. d
11.1.9. d
11.1.10. b

11.1.11. e ($z_2 - z_1$ is the correct answer)
11.1.12. a, b, c, d, e

Chapter 12

12.1. a
12.2. c
12.3. d
12.4. e
12.5. e
12.6. a
12.7. a
12.8. c
12.9. c
12.10. False (only true near the transducer)
12.11. False (only true for normal incidence or oblique incidence when densities and propagation speeds of the media are equal)
12.12. False (see comment for 12.11)
12.13. c
12.14. d
12.15. e (A mode)
12.16. d
12.17. False (6 bits)
12.18. d
12.19. d
12.20. a. 1, 3, 4; b. 2, 5, 6; c. 1, 3, 5
12.21. a
12.22. b
12.23. c
12.24. d (areas are 284 and 3 mm^2)
12.25. c
12.26. d
12.27. e
12.28. c
12.29. d
12.30. d
12.31. c
12.32. c
12.33. b
12.34. Yes
12.35. a
12.36. a
12.37. a
12.38. a
12.39. d (b and c)

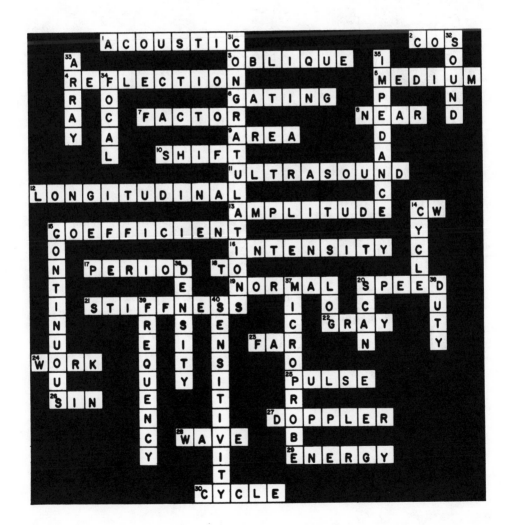

12.40. d

12.41. c

12.42. d

12.43. c

12.44. c

12.45. e (d and a or b)

12.46. a. 1, 2; b. 1, 2; c. 2, 3; d. 1, 2, 3

12.47. c

12.48. b

12.49. b

12.50. c

12.51.

12.52.

DYNAMIC   TWO   GATING

REAL   AMPLIFICATION   INCIDENCE

FAR   PROPAGATION

ECHO   ATTENUATION   WAVE   REFRACTION   VELOCITY

SOUND

TRANSMISSION

CONVERTER   ABSORPTION   INTENSITY

ANECHOIC   DUTY   DOPPLER

LONG   INDEPENDENTLY   IMPEDANCE   SCATTER

GRAY   NORMAL   POWER

MULTIPLE   PULSE   AMPLITUDE

TRANSDUCER   KILO

OBLIQUE   MHZ   ENERGY

LATERAL   FRAME   RAYL

12.53.

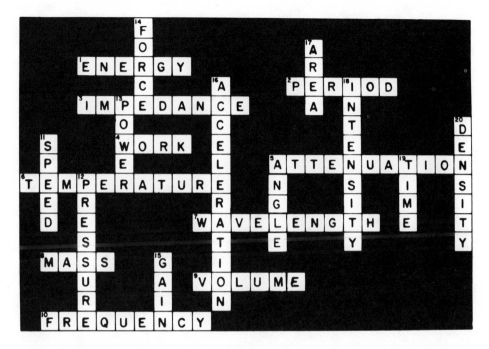

12.54. START

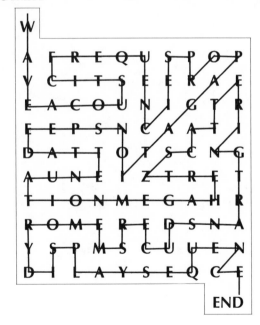

12.55. S

Appendixes

Appendix A
Symbols List

a	attenuation, acceleration
a_C	attenuation coefficient
A	area, current
A_B	beam area
A_P	pressure amplitude
A_v	particle velocity amplitude
ARC	amplitude reflection coefficient
BUR	beam uniformity ratio
BW	bandwidth
c	sound propagation speed
c_m	transducer material propagation speed
d	distance to reflector, displacement
d_m	maximum unambiguous imaging depth
D	half-intensity depth
D_B	beam diameter
D_I	imaging depth
D_T	transducer diameter
DF	duty factor
E	energy
f	frequency
f_i	incident frequency
f_o	operating frequency
f_r	reflected frequency
F	force
FBW	fractional bandwidth
FR	frame rate
I	intensity, current

I_i	incident intensity
I_r	reflected intensity
I_t	transmitted intensity
I_{sa}	spatial average intensity
I_{sp}	spatial peak intensity
I_{TA}	temporal average intensity
I_{TP}	temporal peak intensity
IRC	intensity reflection coefficient
ITC	intensity transmission coefficient
l	path length
LD	line density
LPF	lines per frame
m	mass
M	stiffness
n	number of cycles in a pulse
NZL	near zone length
p	pressure
P	power
PD	pulse duration
PRF	pulse repetition frequency
PRP	pulse repetition period
Q	quality factor
R	resistance
R_A	axial resolution
R_L	lateral resolution
s	speed
S_r	reflector speed
SA	sector angle
SPL	spatial pulse length
t	time, pulse round-trip time
T	period
v	velocity
V	volume, voltage
w	transducer thickness
W	work
W_d	display width
z	impedance
Δf	Doppler shift
Δv	velocity change
ΔV_F	fractional volume change
λ	wavelength
ρ	density
Θ_i	incidence angle
Θ_r	reflection angle
Θ_t	transmission angle

Appendix B
Equations List

For convenient reference, the 40 equations presented throughout this book (excluding Chapter 11 and the appendixes) are compiled here. An asterisk over the equals symbol indicates that the equation is specifically for soft tissues. Two asterisks over the equals symbol indicate that the equation is specifically for perpendicular incidence. The ten most fundamental and important equations are indicated with arrows (⟵).

Chapter 2

$$\text{period } (\mu s) = \frac{1}{\text{frequency (MHz)}} \qquad T = \frac{1}{f}$$

$$\text{wavelength (mm)} = \frac{\text{propagation speed (mm/}\mu s)}{\text{frequency (MHz)}} \qquad \lambda = \frac{c}{f} \quad \longleftarrow$$

$$\text{wavelength (mm)} \overset{*}{=} \frac{1.54}{\text{frequency (MHz)}} \qquad \lambda \overset{*}{=} \frac{1.54}{f}$$

$$\text{impedance (rayl)} = \text{density (kg/m}^3) \times \text{propagation speed (m/s)} \qquad z = \rho c \quad \longleftarrow$$

$$\text{pulse repetition period (ms)} = \frac{1}{\text{pulse repetition frequency (kHz)}} \qquad PRP = \frac{1}{PRF}$$

$$\text{pulse duration (\mu s)} = \text{number of cycles in the pulse} \times \text{period (\mu s)} \qquad PD = n \times T$$

$$\text{pulse duration (\mu s)} = \frac{\text{number of cycles in the pulse}}{\text{frequency (MHz)}} \qquad PD = \frac{n}{f}$$

$$\text{duty factor} = \frac{\text{pulse duration (\mu s)}}{\text{pulse repetition period (ms)} \times 1000} \qquad DF = \frac{PD}{PRP \times 1000} \quad \longleftarrow$$

$$\text{duty factor} = \frac{\text{pulse duration (\mu s)} \times \text{pulse repetition frequency (KHz)}}{1000}$$

$$DF = \frac{PD \times PRF}{1000}$$

$$\text{spatial pulse length (mm)} = \text{number of cycles in the pulse} \times \text{wavelength (mm)} \qquad SPL = n \times \lambda$$

$$\text{spatial pulse length (mm)} = \frac{\text{number of cycles in the pulse} \times \text{propagation speed (mm/\mu s)}}{\text{frequency (MHz)}} \qquad SPL = \frac{n \times c}{f}$$

$$\text{spatial pulse length (mm)} \overset{*}{=} \frac{\text{number of cycles in the pulse} \times 1.54}{\text{frequency (MHz)}} \qquad SPL \overset{*}{=} \frac{n \times 1.54}{f}$$

$$\text{intensity (W/cm}^2) = \frac{\text{power (W)}}{\text{area (cm}^2)} \qquad I = \frac{P}{A} \quad \longleftarrow$$

$$\text{spatial average intensity (W/cm}^2) = \frac{\text{spatial peak intensity (W/cm}^2)}{\text{beam uniformity ratio}} \qquad I_{SA} = \frac{I_{SP}}{BUR}$$

$$\text{temporal average intensity (W/cm}^2) = \text{duty factor} \times \text{temporal peak intensity (W/cm}^2) \qquad I_{TA} = DF \times I_{TP}$$

$$\text{attenuation (dB)} = \text{attenuation coefficient (dB/cm)} \times \text{path length (cm)} \qquad a = a_c\, l$$

$$\text{attenuation (dB)} \overset{*}{=} \text{frequency (MHz)} \times \text{path length (cm)} \qquad a \overset{*}{=} f \times l \quad \longleftarrow$$

$$\text{half-intensity depth (cm)} = \frac{3}{\text{attenuation coefficient (dB/cm)}} \qquad D = \frac{3}{a_c}$$

$$\text{half-intensity depth} \overset{*}{=} \frac{3}{\text{frequency (MHz)}} \qquad D \overset{*}{=} \frac{3}{f}$$

intensity reflection coefficient $= \dfrac{\text{reflected intensity (W/cm}^2)}{\text{incident intensity (W/cm}^2)}$ $IRC = \dfrac{I_r}{I_i}$

$$\overset{..}{=} \left[\dfrac{\text{medium two impedance } - \text{ medium one impedance}}{\text{medium two impedance } + \text{ medium one impedance}}\right]^2 \qquad \overset{..}{=} \left[\dfrac{z_2 - z_1}{z_2 + z_1}\right]^2 \longleftarrow$$

intensity transmission coefficient $= \dfrac{\text{transmitted intensity (W/cm}^2)}{\text{incident intensity (W/cm}^2)}$ $ITC = \dfrac{I_t}{I_i}$

$\overset{..}{=} 1 - $ intensity reflection $\overset{..}{=} 1 - IRC$
coefficient

reflection angle (°) $=$ incidence angle (°) $\theta_r = \theta_i$

transmission angle (°) $=$ incidence angle (°) $\times$

$$\left[\dfrac{\text{medium two propagation speed (mm/}\mu\text{s)}}{\text{medium one propagation speed (mm/}\mu\text{s)}}\right] \quad \theta_t = \theta_i \; \left[\dfrac{c_2}{c_1}\right]$$

distance to reflector (mm) $=$
½ [propagation speed (mm/μs) $\times$ pulse round-trip time (μs)] $d = \frac{1}{2}ct$

distance to reflector (mm) $\overset{*}{=} 0.77 \times$ pulse round-trip time (μs) $d \overset{*}{=} 0.77t \longleftarrow$

---

operating frequency (MHz) $= \dfrac{\text{propagation speed (mm/}\mu\text{s)}}{2 \times \text{thickness (mm)}}$ $f_o = \dfrac{c_m}{2w}$

quality factor $= \dfrac{\text{operating frequency (MHz)}}{\text{bandwidth (MHz)}}$ $Q = \dfrac{f_o}{BW}$

near zone length (mm) $= \dfrac{[\text{transducer diameter (mm)}]^2}{4 \times \text{wavelength (mm)}}$ $NZL = \dfrac{D_T^2}{4\lambda}$

near-zone length (mm) $\overset{*}{=}$
$\dfrac{[\text{transducer diameter (mm)}]^2 \times \text{frequency (MHz)}}{6}$ $NZL \overset{*}{=} \dfrac{D_T^2 f}{6} \longleftarrow$

beam area (cm²) $= 0.8 \times [\text{beam diameter (cm)}]^2$ $A_B = 0.8 \, D_B^2$

axial resolution (mm) $= \dfrac{\text{spatial pulse length (mm)}}{2}$ $R_A = \dfrac{SPL}{2} \longleftarrow$

axial resolution (mm) $\overset{*}{=}$
$\dfrac{0.77 \times \text{number of cycles in the pulse}}{\text{frequency (MHz)}}$ $R_A \overset{*}{=} \dfrac{0.77n}{f}$

lateral resolution (mm) = beam diameter (mm) $R_L = D_B$ ⟵

Chapter 6

pulse repetition frequency (Hz) = lines per frame × frame rate $PRF = LD \times FR$

$$\text{line density (lines/cm)} = \frac{\text{lines per frame}}{\text{display width (cm)}} \qquad LD = \frac{LPF}{W_d}$$

$$\text{line density (lines/degree)} = \frac{\text{lines per frame}}{\text{degrees per sector}} \qquad LD = \frac{LPF}{SA}$$

Chapter 7

Doppler shift (MHz) = reflected frequency (MHz) − incident frequency (MHz)

$$= \pm \frac{2 \times \text{reflector speed (m/s)} \times \text{incident frequency (MHz)}}{\text{propagation speed (m/s)}}$$

$$\Delta f = f_r - f_i = \pm \frac{2 \times S_r \times f_i}{c}$$

Chapter 8

$$\text{maximum depth (cm)} = 77/\text{pulse repetition frequency (kHz)} \qquad d_m = \frac{77}{PRF}$$

pulse repetition frequency (Hz) = lines per frame × frame rate $PRF = LPF \times FR$

maximum depth (cm) × lines per frame × frame rate = 77,000

$$d_m \times LPF \times FR = 77,000$$

Appendix C
Mathematics

Only the basic mathematical concepts that are applicable to the material in this book will be considered in this appendix.

**C.1
Algebra**

Transposition of quantities in algebraic equations is accomplished by performing identical mathematical operations on both sides.

For the equation

*Example
C.1.1.*

$$x + y = z$$

transpose to get x alone (solve for x). To do this, subtract y from both sides:

$$x + y - y = z - y$$

Since $y - y = 0$; the left-hand side of the equation is

$$x + y - y = x + 0 = x$$

so that

$$x = z - y$$

Example C.1.2. For the equation

$$x - y = z$$

solve for x. Add y to both sides:

$$x - y + y = z + y$$
$$x + 0 = z + y$$
$$x = z + y$$

Example C.1.3. For the equation

$$xy = z$$

solve for x. Divide both sides by y:

$$\frac{xy}{y} = \frac{z}{y}$$

Since $\frac{y}{y} = 1$;

$$\frac{xy}{y} = x(1) = x$$

and

$$x = \frac{z}{y}$$

Example C.1.4. For the equation

$$\frac{x}{y} = z$$

solve for x. Multiply both sides by y:

$$\frac{x}{y} y = zy$$
$$x(1) = zy$$
$$x = zy$$

Using some numbers, and combining the previous examples, consider the equation

Example C.1.5.

$$\frac{5x + 3}{2} - 3 = 1$$

Solve for x. Add 3:

$$\frac{5x + 3}{2} - 3 + 3 = 1 + 3$$

$$\frac{5x + 3}{2} = 4$$

Multiply by 2:

$$\frac{5x + 3}{2} \times 2 = 4 \times 2$$

$$5x + 3 = 8$$

Subract 3:

$$5x + 3 - 3 = 8 - 3$$

$$5x = 5$$

Divide by 5:

$$x = 1$$

Substitution of the answer into the original equation shows that the equality is satisfied and the answer is correct:

$$\frac{5(1) + 3}{2} - 3 = 1$$

$$\frac{8}{2} - 3 = 1$$

$$4 - 3 = 1$$

$$1 = 1$$

Example
C.1.6.   For the equation

$$\text{propagation speed} = \text{frequency} \times \text{wavelength}$$

solve for wavelength. Divide by frequency:

$$\frac{\text{propagation speed}}{\text{frequency}} = \frac{\text{frequency} \times \text{wavelength}}{\text{frequency}}$$

$$\frac{\text{propagaton speed}}{\text{frequency}} = \text{wavelength}$$

Example
C.1.7.   If the intensity reflection coefficient is 0.1 and the reflected intensity is 5 mW/cm², find the incident intensity, given that

$$\text{intensity reflection coefficient} = \frac{\text{reflected intensity}}{\text{incident intensity}}$$

Multiply by incident intensity:

$$\text{intensity reflection coefficient} \times \text{incident intensity}$$
$$= \frac{\text{reflected intensity}}{\text{incident intensity}} \times \text{incident intensity} = \text{reflected intensity}$$

Divide by intensity reflection coefficient:

$$\frac{\text{intensity reflection coefficient} \times \text{incident intensity}}{\text{intensity reflection coefficient}}$$

$$= \frac{\text{reflected intensity}}{\text{intensity reflection coefficient}}$$

$$\text{incident intensity} = \frac{\text{reflected intensity}}{\text{intensity reflection coefficient}}$$

$$= \frac{5 \text{ mW/cm}^2}{0.1}$$

$$= 50 \text{ mW/cm}^2$$

Example
C.1.8.   If the intensity reflection coefficient is 0.01 and the impedance for medium one is 4.5, find the medium two impedance, given that

$$\text{intensity reflection coefficient} =$$

$$\left[\frac{\text{medium two impedance} - \text{medium one impedance}}{\text{medium two impedance} + \text{medium one impedance}} \right]^2$$

Take the square root of each side:

$$\text{(intensity reflection coefficient)}^{1/2} = \frac{\text{medium two impedance} - \text{medium one impedance}}{\text{medium two impedance} + \text{medium one impedance}}$$

Multiply by the sum of medium two impedance and medium one impedance:

$$\text{(intensity reflection coefficient)}^{1/2} \times$$
$$\text{(medium two impedance} + \text{medium one impedance)} =$$
$$\text{medium two impedance} - \text{medium one impedance}$$

Add the medium one impedance:

$$\text{(intensity reflection coefficient)}^{1/2} \times$$
$$\text{(medium two impedance} + \text{medium one impedance)} +$$
$$\text{medium one impedance} = \text{medium two impedance}$$

Subtract (intensity reflection coefficient)$^{1/2}$ × medium two impedance:

$$[\text{(intensity reflection coefficient)}^{1/2} \times \text{medium one impedance]}$$
$$+ \text{medium one impedance} = \text{medium two impedance}$$
$$- [\text{(intensity reflection coefficient)}^{1/2} \times \text{medium two impedance]}$$

$$\text{medium one impedance } [1 + \text{(intensity reflection coefficient)}^{1/2}]$$
$$= \text{medium two impedance } [1 - \text{(intensity reflection coefficient)}^{1/2}]$$

Divide by $[1 - \text{(intensity reflection coefficient)}^{1/2}]$ and interchange sides of the equation:

$$\text{medium two impedance} = \text{medium one impedance}$$
$$\left[\frac{1 + \text{(intensity reflection coefficient)}^{1/2}}{1 - \text{(intensity reflection coefficient)}^{1/2}}\right]$$
$$= 4.5 \left[\frac{1 + (0.01)^{1/2}}{1 - (0.01)^{1/2}}\right]$$
$$= 4.5 \left[\frac{1 + 0.1}{1 - 0.1}\right] = 4.5 \left[\frac{1.1}{0.9}\right]$$
$$= 4.5 \ (1.22) = 5.5$$
$$\text{medium two impedance} = 5.5$$

Example
C.1.9.
A sonographer is twice as old as her diagnostic instrument was when she was as old as it is now. She is 24 years old. How old is the instrument? Let x = the instrument's present age. Let y = the instrument's age when the sonographer's age was x. The sonographer's present age is 24 = 2y. Let z = years since the sonographer's age was x and the instrument's age was y. From the information given, we have

$$y + z = x$$

$$x + z = 24$$

$$2y = 24$$

Now solve these three equations for x:

$$y = 24/2 = 12$$

$$z = 24 - x$$

$$x = y + z = 12 + 24 - x$$

$$2x = 36$$

$$x = 18$$

The instrument is 18 years old. It is time to replace the instrument, but not the sonographer.

Exercises

C.1.1. Solve each of the following for x:
a. $x + y + 2 = z$
b. $x - y = z - 1$
c. $2xy = z$
d. $x/y = 3z$
e. $\dfrac{x + 5}{4} - 2 = 4$
f. $\dfrac{3x + 3}{2} - 2 = 4$

C.1.2. Solve each of the following for the quantity with the asterisk:
a. propagation speed = frequency* × wavelength
b. intensity $= \dfrac{\text{power}}{\text{beam area*}}$
c. period $= \dfrac{1}{\text{frequency*}}$

C.1.3. What are the present ages of the following sonographers? Sam was one when Sue was twice as old as Sal. Sue was seven when Sam was half as old as Sal. Their present ages total 79.

C.1.4. The age of an ultrasound instrument is three times its age three years from now minus three times its age three years ago. What is its present age?

C.1.5. Let:

$$y + x = \frac{1}{2}(7y - 3x)$$

Subtract 2x from both sides so that:

$$y - x = \frac{1}{2}(7y - 3x) - 2x$$

Divide both sides by (y − x):

$$\frac{y - x}{y - x} = \frac{7y - 3x}{2(y - x)} - \frac{2x}{y - x}$$

Combine right side into single fraction:

$$\frac{y - x}{y - x} = \frac{7y - 3x - 4x}{2(y - x)} = \frac{7(y - x)}{2(y - x)}$$

Multiply both sides by 2:

$$2\left[\frac{y - x}{y - x}\right] = 7\left[\frac{y - x}{y - x}\right]$$

Therefore, 2 = 7. What went wrong?

If the sides and angles of a right triangle (one of the angles equals 90 degrees) are labeled as in Figure C.1, the **sine** of angle A (**sin** A) and the cosine of angle A (cos A) are defined as follows:

C.2

Trigonometry

$$\sin A = \frac{\text{length of side a}}{\text{length of side c}}$$

$$\cos A = \frac{\text{length of side b}}{\text{length of side c}}$$

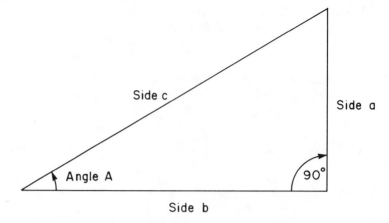

Figure C.1. Sides and angles of a right triangle.

Example
C.2.1
If the lengths of sides a, b, and c are 1, $\sqrt{3}$, and 2, respectively, what are sin A and cos A?

$$\sin A = \frac{1}{2} = 0.50$$

$$\cos A = \frac{\sqrt{3}}{2} = 0.87$$

If the sine or cosine is known, angle A may be found using a calculator or a table such as Table C.1.

Table C.1
Sines and Cosines for Various Angles

Angle A (degrees)	sin A	cos A
0	0.00	1.00
1	0.02	1.00
2	0.03	1.00
3	0.05	1.00
4	0.07	1.00
5	0.09	1.00
6	0.10	0.99
7	0.12	0.99
8	0.14	0.99
9	0.16	0.99
10	0.17	0.98
20	0.34	0.94
30	0.50	0.87
40	0.64	0.77
50	0.77	0.64
60	0.87	0.50
70	0.94	0.34
80	0.98	0.17
90	1.00	0.00

If sin A is 0.5, what is A? From Table C.1, A = 30 degrees.

Example
C.2.2

If cos A is 0.87, what is A? From Table C.1, A = 30 degrees.
  If angle A is known, sin A or cos A may be found using a calculator or a table such as Table C.3.1.

Example
C.2.3

If A = 40 degrees ,what are sin A and cos A? From Table C.1, sin A = 0.64 and cos A = 0.77.

Example
C.2.4

Exercises

C.2.1. If sides a, b, and c in Figure C.1 have lengths 3, 4, and 5, respectively, sin A is _____ and cos A is _____ .

C.2.2. If angle A is 90 degrees, sin A is _____ and cos A is _____ .

C.2.3. If sin A is 0.17, angle A is _____ degrees.

C.2.4. If cos A is 0.94, angle A is _____ degrees.

The **logarithm** (**log**) (to the base 10) of a number is equal to the number of tens that must be multiplied together to result in that number. More generally, it is the power to which 10 must be raised to give a particular number.

**C.3
Logarithms
and
Scientific
Notation**

What is the logarithm of 1000? To obtain 1000, three tens must be multiplied together:

Example
C.3.1

$$10 \times 10 \times 10 = 1000$$

Three tens then yield the logarithm (log) of 1000.

$$\log 1000 = 3$$

The logarithm of the reciprocal of a number is equal to the negative of the logarithm of the number.

Example
C.3.2 What is the logarithm of 0.01?

$$0.01 = \frac{1}{100}$$

$$\log 100 = 2$$

$$\log 0.01 = \log \frac{1}{100} = -2$$

Scientific notation is a means of compactly expressing numbers (especially very large or very small ones). It makes use of logarithms or powers of ten as follows. The log of 100,000 is 5, i.e., 100,000 = 10^5 so the number, 100,000, may be expressed as 1×10^5. The log of .000000001 $\left(\dfrac{1}{1,000,000,000}\right)$ is -9. Therefore it may be expressed as 1×10^{-9}.

Example
C.3.3 Here are several numbers expressed in scientific notation:

500	5×10^2
531,000,000	5.31×10^8
10	1×10^1
1	1×10^0
.00052	5.2×10^{-4}
.0000001	1×10^{-7}

Exercises

C.3.1. Give the logarithms of the following numbers:
   a. 10 _____
   b. 0.1 _____
   c. 100 _____
   d. 0.001 _____

C.3.2. Express the following in scientific notation:
   a. 55,000 _____
   b. 422,000,000 _____
   c. .005 _____
   d. .000000082 _____

C.4
Decibels Decibels are units that result from taking 10 times the logarithm of the ratio of two powers or intensities.

Compare the following two powers in decibels: power one = 1 W; power two = 10 W.

Example C.4.1

$$10 \log \frac{\text{power one}}{\text{power two}} = 10 \log \frac{1}{10}$$

$$= 10 \left(-\log 10\right) = 10 \left(-1\right) = -10 \text{ dB}$$

Power one is 10 dB less than power two, or power one is 10 dB below power two. Also

$$10 \log \frac{\text{power two}}{\text{power one}} = 10 \log \frac{10}{1}$$

$$= 10 \left(\log 10\right) = 10 \left(1\right) = 10 \text{ dB}$$

Power two is 10 dB more than power one, or power two is 10 dB above power one.

An amplifier has a power output of 100 mW when the input power is 0.1 mW. What is the amplifier gain in decibels?

Example C.4.2

$$\text{amplifier gain (db)} = 10 \log \frac{\text{power out}}{\text{power in}}$$

$$= 10 \log \frac{100}{0.1} = 10 \log 1000 = 10 \left(3\right) = 30 \text{ dB}$$

An electric attenuator has a power output of 0.01 mW when the input power is 100 mW. What is the attenuator attenuation in decibels?

Example C.4.3

$$\text{attenuator attenuation (dB)} = - 10 \log \frac{\text{power out}}{\text{power in}}$$

$$= - 10 \log \frac{0.01}{100} = - 10 \log \frac{1}{10,000}$$

$$= - 10 \left(-\log 10,000\right) = - 10 \left(-4\right) = 40 \text{ dB}$$

The first minus sign is used here to give the attenuation as a positive number. If the minus number had not been used, the "gain" of the attenuator would have been calculated, which would have turned out to be -40 dB. A gain of -40 dB is the same as an attenuation of 40 dB.

Example
C.4.4

Compare intensity two with intensity one: intensity one $= 10$ mW/cm^2; intensity two $= 0.01$ mW/cm^2.

$$10 \log \frac{\text{intensity two}}{\text{intensity one}} = 10 \log \frac{0.01}{10}$$

$$= 10 \log \frac{1}{1000} = 10 \, (-\log 1000) = 10 \, (-3) = -30 \text{ dB}$$

Intensity two is 30 dB less than or below intensity one.

Example
C.4.5

As sound passes through a medium, its intensity at one point is 1 mW/cm^2 and at a point 10 cm farther along is 0.1 mW/cm^2. What are the attenuation and attenuation coefficient? (See Section 2.5.)

$$\text{attenuation (dB)} = -10 \log \frac{\text{intensity at second point}}{\text{intensity at first point}}$$

$$= -10 \log \frac{0.1}{1} = -10 \log \frac{1}{10} = -10 \, (-\log 10)$$

$$= -10 \, (-1) = 10 \text{ dB}$$

See Example C.4.3 for comment on the first minus sign. The attenuation coefficient is the attenuation (dB) divided by the separation between the two points:

$$\text{attenuation coefficient (dB/cm)} = \frac{\text{attenuation (dB)}}{\text{separation (cm)}}$$

$$= \frac{10 \text{ dB}}{10 \text{ cm}} = 1 \text{ dB/cm}$$

Table C.2 lists various values of power or intensity ratio with corresponding decibel values of gain or attenuation.

Table C.2
Decibel Values of Gain or Attenuation for Various
Values of Power or Intensity Ratio*

| dB Gain or attenuation | Intensity or Power Ratio | |
	Attenuation	Gain
1	.79	1.3
2	.63	1.6
3	.50	2.0
4	.40	2.5
5	.32	3.2
6	.25	4.0
7	.20	5.0
8	.16	6.3
9	.13	7.9
10	.10	10.0
15	.032	32.0
20	.01	100.0
25	.003	320.0
30	.001	1,000.0
35	.0003	3,200.0
40	.0001	10,000.0
45	.00003	32,000.0
50	.00001	100,000.0
60	.000001	1,000,000.0
70	.0000001	10,000,000.0
80	.00000001	100,000,000.0
90	.000000001	1,000,000,000.0
100	.0000000001	10,000,000,000.0

*The ratio is output power or intensity divided by input power or intensity. In the case of attenuation, it is the fraction of power or intensity remaining.

Some authors always put output or end-of-path values in the numerator of the equation used for calculating decibels. If the numerator value is less than the denominator value (e.g., attenuation) a negative decibel value is calculated. For example, if the input and output powers for an electrical attenuator were 2 and 1 W, respectively, -3 dB results. That is, this attenuator has -3 dB of gain. In this book, only positive dB values are considered. In the example, the result would be given as 3 dB of attenuation.

Exercises

C.4.1. One watt is _____ dB below 100 W.

C.4.2. One watt is _____ dB above 100 mW.

C.4.3. If the input power is 1 mW and the output is 10,000 mW, the gain is _____ dB.

C.4.4. If the input power is 1 W and the output is 100 mW, the gain is _____ dB. The attenuation is _____ dB.

C.4.5. If the intensities of traveling sound are 10 mW/cm^2 and 0.1 mW/cm^2 at two points 5 cm apart, the attenuation between the two points is _____ dB. The attenuation coefficient is _____ dB/cm.

C.4.6. If an amplifier has a gain of 15 dB, the ratio of output power to input power is _____. (Use Table C.2.)

C.4.7. If an attenuator has an attenuation of 25 dB, the ratio of output power to input power is _____. (Use Table C.2.)

C.4.8. If the intensity at the start of a path is 3 mW/cm^2 and the attenuation over the path is 2 dB, the intensity at the end of the path is _____ mW/cm^2. (Use Table C.2)

C.4.9. If the output of a 22-dB gain amplifier is connected to the input of a 23-dB gain amplifier, the total gain is _____ dB. The overall power ratio is _____. (Use Table C.2.)

C.4.10. If a 17-dB attenuator is connected to a 15-dB amplifier, the net gain is _____ dB. The net attenuation is _____ dB. For a 1-W input, the output is _____ W. (Use Table C.2.)

C.5 Binary Numbers

The use of digital memories in ultrasound imaging instruments (Section 5.4) presents a need for understanding the binary-numbering system. Digital (computer) memories and data processors use binary numbers in carrying out their functions. This is because they contain electronic components that operate in only two states, off (0) and on (1).

Binary digits (bits) consist of only zeros and ones, represented by the symbols 0 and 1. As in the decimal numbering system, with which we are so familiar, other numbers must be represented by moving these symbols to different positions (columns). In the decimal system, where there are ten symbols (0 through 9), there is no symbol for the number ten (nine is the largest number for which there is a symbol). To represent ten in symbolic form, the symbol for one is used but moved to the second (from the right) column. A zero is placed in the right column to clarify this so that ten is, symbolically, 10. The symbol for one has been used but in such a way that it no longer represents one, but, rather, ten.

A similar procedure is used in the binary numbering system. The symbol 1 represents the largest number (one) for which there is a symbol in the system. To represent the next number (two), the same thing is done as in the decimal system. That is, the symbol 1 is placed in the next column to represent the number two.

Columns in the two systems represent values as follows:

decimal:

millions	hundred-thousands	ten-thousands	thousands	hundreds	tens	ones

binary:

sixty-fours	thirty-twos	sixteens	eights	fours	twos	ones

In the decimal system, each column represents ten times the column to the right. In the binary system each column represents two times the column to the right.

The decimal number, 1234, represents (reading from right to left) four ones, three tens, two hundreds, and one thousand, i.e., $4 + 30 + 200 + 1000 = 1,234$. The *decimal* number, 10110, represents zero ones, one ten, one hundred, zero thousands, and one ten thousand. The *binary* number, 10110, represents zero ones, one two, one four, zero eights, and one sixteen, i.e., $0 + 2 + 4 + 0 + 16 = 22$ (in decimal form). The previous sentence represents a straightforward way of converting a number from binary to decimal. To convert from decimal to binary, repeated division by two is used as follows. Divide the decimal number by two and note the remainder. Divide the quotient (from the previous division) by two and note the remainder. Continue until the quotient is zero. Write the remainders from first to last in order from right to left, respectively, to get the binary number equivalent of the initial decimal number.

Convert the decimal number 60 to binary:

Example C.5.1

		quotient	remainder
2)60	=	30	0
2)30	=	15	0
2)15	=	7	1
2)7	=	3	1
2)3	=	1	1
2)1	=	0	1

The binary form of 60 is, therefore, 111100.

Example C.5.2. Convert the binary number 101010 to decimal form. This number represents $0 + 2 + 0 + 8 + 0 + 32 = 42$ in decimal. To check this answer, convert 42 back to binary.

			quotient	remainder
2)42	=		21	0
2)21	=		10	1
2)10	=		5	0
2)5	=		2	1
2)2	=		1	0
2)1	=		0	1

i.e., 101010.

Table C.3 lists the binary forms of the decimal numbers 0 through 63.

Table C.3
Binary and Decimal Number Equivalents

Decimal	Binary	Decimal	Binary
0	000000	32	100000
1	000001	33	100001
2	000010	34	100010
3	000011	35	100011
4	000100	36	100100
5	000101	37	100101
6	000110	38	100110
7	000111	39	100111
8	001000	40	101000
9	001001	41	101001
10	001010	42	101010
11	001011	43	101011
12	001100	44	101100
13	001101	45	101101
14	001110	46	101110
15	001111	47	101111
16	010000	48	110000
17	010001	49	110001
18	010010	50	110010
19	010011	51	110011
20	010100	52	110100
21	010101	53	110101
22	010110	54	110110
23	010111	55	110111
24	011000	56	111000
25	011001	57	111001
26	011010	58	111010
27	011011	59	111011
28	011100	60	111100
29	011101	61	111101
30	011110	62	111110
31	011111	63	111111

C.5.1. In binary numbers, how many symbols are used? _____

C.5.2. The term "binary digit" is commonly shortened into the single word _____ .

C.5.3. Each binary digit in a binary number is represented in memory by a memory element, which at any time is in one of _____ states.

C.5.4. Match the following:

Column in a binary number   Decimal number represented
hgfedcba   by a 1 in the column

a. _____   1. 64
b. _____   2. 32
c. _____   3. 1
d. _____   4. 16
e. _____   5. 8
f. _____   6. 128
g. _____   7. 2
h. _____   8. 4

C.5.5. The binary number 10110 represents zero ones, one two, one four, zero eights, and one sixteen, i.e., $0 + 2 + 4 + 0 + 16 = 22$. What decimal number is represented by the binary number 11001? _____

C.5.6. The decimal number 13 is made up of one one, zero twos, one four, and one eight ($8 + 4 + 0 + 1 = 13$). It is therefore represented by the binary number _____ .

C.5.7. Match the following

a. 1 _____   1. 0001111
b. 5 _____   2. 0011001
c. 10 _____   3. 0001010
d. 15 _____   4. 0110010
e. 20 _____   5. 0000001
f. 25 _____   6. 1100100
g. 30 _____   7. 0101000
h. 40 _____   8. 0011110
i. 50 _____   9. 0010100
j. 100 _____   10. 0000101

C.5.8. How many binary digits are required in the binary numbers representing the following decimal numbers?

a. 0 _____
b. 1 _____
c. 5 _____
d. 10 _____
e. 25 _____

f. 30 _____
g. 63 _____
h. 64 _____
i. 75 _____
j. 100 _____

C.5.9. Match the following:

Largest decimal number that can be represented	by a binary number with this many bits
a. 7 _____	1. 1
b. 15 _____	2. 2
c. 3 _____	3. 3
d. 511 _____	4. 4
e. 1023 _____	5 .5
f. 63 _____	6. 6
g. 255 _____	7. 7
h. 1 _____	8. 8
i. 127 _____	9. 9
j. 31 _____	10. 10

C.5.10. How many bits are required to store numbers representing each number of different gray shades?

a.   2 _____
b.   4 _____
c.   8 _____
d.   15 _____
e.   16 _____
f.   25 _____
g.   32 _____
h.   64 _____
i.   65 _____
j. 128 _____

C.6 Units

Units for the physics and acoustics quantities discussed in this book are presented in this appendix. They are drawn primarily from the international system of units (SI).

Units for the quantities discussed in this book are listed in Table C.4. Equivalent units are given in Table C.5. Prefixes for units are listed in Table C.6, and conversion factors between common units are in Table C.7.

In algebraic equations involving these units, the units for the quantity solved for are determined by manipulation of the units for the other quantities in the equation.

Table C.4

Units and Unit Symbols for Physics and Acoustics Quantities

Quantity	Unit	Unit symbol
Acceleration	meters/second^2	m/s^2
Angle	degrees	degrees
Area	meters^2	m^2
Attenuation	decibels	dB
Attenuation coefficient	decibels/meter	dB/m
Beam area	meters^2	m^2
Beam uniformity ratio	unitless	—
Cosine	unitless	—
Current	amperes	A
Density	kilograms/meter^3	kg/m^3
Displacement	meters	m
Doppler shift	hertz	Hz
Duty factor	unitless	—
Energy	joules	J
Force	newtons	N
Fractional volume change	unitless	—
Frequency	hertz	Hz
Gain	decibels	dB
Half-intensity depth	meters	m
Heat	joules	J
Impedance	rayls	—
Intensity	watts/meters^2	W/m^2
Intensity reflection coefficient	unitless	—
Intensity transmission coefficient	unitless	—
Mass	kilograms	kg
Period	seconds	s
Power	watts	W
Pressure	newtons/meter^2	N/m^2
Propagation speed	meters/second	m/s
Pulse duration	seconds	s
Pulse repetition frequency	hertz	Hz
Pulse repetition period	seconds	s
Resistance	ohms	Ω
Sine	unitless	—
Spatial pulse length	meters	m
Speed	meters/second	m/s
Stiffness	newtons/meter^2	N/m^2
Temperature	kelvins	K
Time	seconds	s
Velocity	meters/second	m/s
Voltage	volts	V
Volume	meters^3	m^3
Wavelength	meters	m
Work	joules	J

Table C.5

Equivalent Units for Physics and Acoustics Quantities

Unit given in Table C.4	Equivalent unit	Equivalent unit symbol
Hertz	1/second	1/s
Joules	newton-meters	N-m
Joules	watt-seconds	W-s
Rayls	kilograms/meter^2-second	kg/m^2-s
Newtons	kilogram-meters/second^2	kg-m/s^2
Newtons/meter^2	pascals	Pa
Watts	joules/second	J/s

Table C.6

Unit Prefixes

Prefix	Factor*	Symbol
mega	1,000,000	M
kilo	1,000	k
centi	0.01	c
milli	0.001	m
micro	0.000001	μ

*Factor is the number of unprefixed units in a unit with the prefix. For example, there are 1,000 Hz in 1 kHz, and there is 0.001 m in 1 mm.

Table C.7

Conversion Factors among Common Units

To convert	from	to	multiply by
Area	m^2	cm^2	10,000
	cm^2	m^2	0.0001
Attenuation	dB	Np (neper)	0.12
Displacement	m	mm	1,000
	m	cm	100
	m	km	0.001
	mm	m	0.001
	mm	km	0.000001
	km	mm	1,000,000
Frequency	Hz	kHz	0.001
	Hz	MHz	0.000001
	kHz	MHz	0.001
	MHz	kHz	1,000
	kHz	Hz	1,000
	MHz	Hz	1,000,000
Intensity	W/cm^2	W/m^2	10,000
	W/cm^2	kW/m^2	10
	W/cm^2	mW/cm^2	1,000
	W/m^2	W/cm^2	0.0001
	W/m^2	mW/cm^2	0.1
	W/m^2	kW/m^2	0.001
Speed	m/s	km/s	0.001
	km/s	m/s	1,000
	km/s	mm/μs	1

Determine the unit for frequency in the equation

Example C.6.1

$$\text{frequency} = \frac{\text{propagation speed (m/s)}}{\text{wavelength (m)}}$$

The units on the right-hand side of the equation are

$$\frac{\text{m/s}}{\text{m}} = 1/\text{s}$$

From Table C.5, it can be found that

$$1/\text{s} = \text{Hz}$$

Therefore the frequency unit is hertz.

Determine the unit for frequency in the equation

Example C.6.2

$$\text{frequency} = \frac{\text{propagation speed (m/s)}}{\text{wavelength (mm)}}$$

The units on the right-hand side of the equation are

$$\frac{\text{m/s}}{\text{mm}}$$

From Table C.6, it can be found that 1 mm equals 0.001 m, so that

$$\frac{\text{m/s}}{0.001 \text{ m}} = 1000 \ 1/\text{s}$$

and from Tables C.5 and C.6,

$$1000 \ 1/\text{s} = 1000 \text{ Hz} = 1 \text{ kHz}$$

Therefore the frequency unit is kilohertz. To convert a frequency given in kilohertz to megahertz, multiply by 0.001. To convert a frequency given in kilohertz to hertz, multiply by 1000.

Determine the unit for intensity in the equation

Example C.6.3

$$\text{intensity} = \frac{\text{power (W)}}{\text{area (cm}^2)}$$

The units on the right-hand side of the equation are

$$\frac{W}{cm^2}$$

Therefore the intensity unit is watts per centimeter squared.

Example C.6.4 Determine the unit for impedance in the equation

$$impedance = density\ (kg/m^3) \times propagation\ speed\ (km/s)$$

The units on the right-hand side of the equation are

$$\frac{kg}{m^3} \times \frac{km}{s}$$

From Table C.6,

$$\frac{kg}{m^3} \times \frac{km}{s} = \frac{kg}{m^3} \times \frac{1000\ m}{s} = 1000\ \frac{kg}{m^2\text{-}s}$$

From Table C.5,

$$1000\ \frac{kg}{m^2\text{-}s} = 1000\ rayl$$

From Table C.6,

$$1000\ rayl = 1\ krayl$$

Therefore the impedance unit is kilorayl. Since this is uncommon, it would be better to multiply the answer by 1000 to give the result in rayls.

Exercises

C.6.1. The unit of frequency in the equation

$$frequency = \frac{propagation\ speed\ (km/s)}{wavelength\ (mm)}$$

is _____ . To convert frequency in this unit to frequency in kilohertz, multiply by _____ .

C.6.2. A frequency of 50 kHz is equal to _____ MHz and _____ Hz.

C.6.3. A speed of 1.5 mm/µs is equal to _____ km/s, _____ m/s, _____ cm/s, and _____ mm/s.

C.6.4. If the frequency is 2 MHz and

$$\text{period} = \frac{1}{\text{frequency}}$$

the period is _____ µs, _____ ms, or _____ s.

C.6.5. Mass is given in units of
a. megahertz
b. kilogram
c. telegram
d. millinery
e. none of the above

C.6.6. Displacement is given in
a. megahertz
b. megaphone
c. centipede
d. meter
e. all of the above

C.6.7. Attenuation is given in
a. decimal
b. decimate
c. decibel
d. decimeter
e. decihertz

Appendix D
Physics Concepts

The terms discussed in this appendix are defined in the Glossary. Their units are given in Appendix C. The definitions are amplified here and the terms are related to one another.

D.1
Mechanics

If there were no **forces,** everything would be in a state of rest or steady motion. Forces change the state of rest or motion of matter. When considering sound, the force divided by the area over which the force is applied is a useful quantity. This is called pressure, one of the acoustic variables discussed in Chapter 2. It is force per unit area (the concentration of force).

$$\text{pressure (N/m}^2) = \frac{\text{force (N)}}{\text{area (m}^2)} \qquad p = \frac{F}{A}$$

A given force applied to an object may produce markedly different results if the pressures at which it is applied are different. If, for example, a small force is applied by a hand to an inflated toy balloon, the balloon will simply move. If the same small force is applied by a sharp needle, the balloon will break. The difference is that the needle applies the force over a very small area (a very high pressure), breaking the balloon.

Application of force or pressure changes the state of rest or motion of matter. Motion may be described in many ways.

Displacement is the distance that a body has moved.

Speed is the rate at which position is changing. It is the distance moved divided by the time over which the movement occurs.

$$\text{speed (m/s)} = \frac{\text{displacement (m)}}{\text{time (s)}} \qquad s = \frac{d}{t}$$

Velocity is the same as speed except that the direction of motion is specified.

Acceleration is the rate at which velocity is changing. It is the change in velocity (change in speed or direction or both) divided by the time over which the change occurs.

$$\text{acceleration (m/s}^2) = \frac{\text{velocity change (m/s)}}{\text{time (s)}} \qquad a = \frac{\Delta v}{t}$$

Mass is a measure of an object's resistance to acceleration. Weight is the gravitational force between two bodies attracting each other. The mass of a body is the same whether it is on the earth or on the moon, but the weights of the body in the two places are quite different.

Density is the concentration of mass. It is the mass divided by the volume taken up by the mass (mass per unit volume).

$$\text{density (kg/m}^3) = \frac{\text{mass (kg)}}{\text{volume (m}^3)} \qquad \rho = \frac{m}{v}$$

Stiffness is a description of the resistance of a material to compression. It is equal to the applied pressure divided by the fractional change in volume resulting from the pressure.

$$\text{stiffness (N/m}^2) = \frac{\text{pressure (N/m}^2)}{\text{fractional volume change}} \qquad M = \frac{p}{\Delta V_F}$$

The fractional volume change is the difference in volume before and after the pressure is applied, divided by the volume before the pressure is applied.

If a material has high stiffness, little change in volume will occur when pressure is applied. If it has low stiffness, a large change in volume will occur when pressure is applied. Stiffness is also called bulk modulus of elasticity. It is equal to the reciprocal of the **compressibility** of a material.

Newton's second law of motion relates three of the things discussed in this appendix. It says that the force applied to a body is equal to the mass of the body multiplied by the acceleration of the body resulting from the applied force.

$$\text{force (N)} = \text{mass (kg)} \times \text{acceleration (m/s}^2) \quad F = ma$$

If more than one force is applied, the net force (resulting from combination of the applied forces) is the force used in the equation. The acceleration will always be in the direction of the net force.

Exercises

D.1.1. To convert speed to velocity, _____ must be specified.

D.1.2. Increased mass results in _____ weight.

D.1.3. Pressure is the concentration of _____ .

D.1.4. Density is the concentration of _____ .

D.1.5. Speed is the rate at which _____ changes.

D.1.6. Acceleration is the rate at which _____ changes.

D.1.7. Newton's second law of motion states that _____ equals _____ times _____ .

D.1.8. Stiffness is a description of the resistance of a material to _____ .

D.1.9. If a force of 50 N acts uniformly over an area of 20 m^2, the pressure is _____ N/m^2.

D.1.10. If a body moves 50 m uniformly in 5 s, its speed is _____ m/s.

D.1.11. If a body accelerates uniformly to the east at 5 m/s^2, its velocity 5 s after the starting from zero speed is _____ m/s east.

D.1.12. Five kilograms of matter with a volume of 10 m^3 have a density of _____ kg/m^3.

D.1.13. If a pressure of 5 N/m^2 changes the volume of a body from 0.5 m^3 to 0.4 m^3, the fractional volume change is _____ .

D.1.14. The stiffness of the material of the body in Problem D.1.13 is _____ N/m^2.

D.1.15. A 5-kg mass subjected to a 15-N force west will have acceleration of _____ m/s² in the _____ direction.

Work is done when a force acts against a resistance to produce motion of a body. It is equal to the applied net force multiplied by the distance the body moves (displacement).

work (J) = force (N) × displacement (m)	W = Fd

If there is no motion, no work is done. If a body is in motion but no force is being applied, no work is done.

Energy is the capability of doing work. A body must have energy in order to do work on another body. When a body does work, it loses energy. When a body has work done on it, it receives energy. Work may be thought of as the transfer of energy from one body (the one doing the work) to another (the one having work done on it). The energy transferred is equal to the work done.

Power is the rate at which work is done or the rate at which energy is transferred. It is equal to the work done divided by the time required to do the work. It is also equal to energy transferred divided by the time required to transfer the energy.

$$\text{power (W)} = \frac{\text{work (J)}}{\text{time (s)}} = \frac{\text{energy (J)}}{\text{time (s)}} \qquad P = \frac{W}{t} = \frac{E}{t}$$

Heat is one type of energy. It is the energy resulting from thermal molecular motion.

Temperature is the condition of a body that determines transfer of heat to or from other bodies. No heat flows when two bodies of equal temperatures come in contact with each other. Heat flows from a body of higher temperature to one of lower temperature when they come in contact.

Electricity is another type of energy. It is the energy resulting from the displacement or flow of electrons. Electric voltage is the work done when moving a unit electric charge between two points across which the voltage exists. It is measured in volts. **Electric current** is the rate of flow of electrons in an electrical conductor. This flow is caused by a voltage. Electric current is measured in amperes. The quantity of current is determined not only by the voltage but also by the **electric resistance** of the conductor. Ohm's law relates voltage, current, and resistance.

| voltage (V) = current (A) × resistance (Ω) | V = I × R |

Electric power is equal to voltage multiplied by current.

| power (W) = voltage (V) × current (A) | P = V × A |

Combining Ohm's law and the electric power equation yields:

| power (W) = current² (A²) × resistance (Ω) | P = I² × R |
| $= \dfrac{\text{voltage}^2 (V^2)}{\text{resistance } (\Omega)}$ | $= \dfrac{V^2}{R}$ |

Exercises

D.2.1. Match the following:

a. pressure: _____   1. force × displacement
b. speed: _____   2. displacement change/time
c. acceleration: _____   3. mass × acceleration
d. density: _____   4. work/time
e. force _____   5. force/area
f. stiffness: _____   6. velocity change/time
g. work: _____   7. mass/volume
h. power: _____   8. pressure/fractional volume
i. electric power: _____   change
j. voltage: _____   9. current × resistance
                              10. voltage × current

D.2.2. Power is the rate at which _____ is done.

D.2.3. Energy is the capability of doing _____ .

D.2.4. Temperature is the condition of a body that determines transfer of _____ to or from other bodies.

D.2.5. Heat and electricity are two types of _____ .

D.2.6. If the current is 2 amperes and the resistance is 12 ohms, the voltage is _____ V and the power is _____ W.

D.2.7. If the current is 25 mA and the resistance is 50 kΩ, the voltage is _____ V and the power is _____ W.

D.2.8. If current is doubled (constant resistance), voltage is _____ and power is _____ .

D.2.9. If resistance is doubled (constant current), voltage is _____ and power is _____ .

D.2.10. Ohm's law relates _____ , _____ , and _____ .

D.2.11. Voltage times current equals electric _____ .

D.2.12. Electric power equals (3 correct answers)
   a. current × resistance
   b. current × voltage
   c. voltage × resistance
   d. current^2 × resistance
   e. voltage^2 ÷ resistance

D.2.13. For 10 volts and 5 amperes, the power is _____ W.

D.2.14. For 10 ohms and 5 amperes, the voltage is _____ V.

D.2.15. If a force of 3 N moves a body 4 m, the work done is _____ J.

D.2.16. If the movement in Problem D.2.15 occurs in 6 s, the power is _____ J/s or _____ W.

D.2.17. In Problem D.2.15, the energy transferred is _____ J.

Answers to Exercises in the Appendixes

Appendix C **C.1.1.** a. $z - y - 2$; b. $y + z - 1$; c. $z/2y$; d. $3yz$; e. 19; f. 3

C.1.2. a. propagation speed/wavelength; b. power/intensity; c. 1/period

C.1.3. Sam is 24, Sal is 26, and Sue is 29.

C.1.4. 18

C.1.5. Division by zero is what went wrong.
Note that

$$y + x = \frac{1}{2}(7y - 3x)$$

yields

$$2(y + x) = 7y - 3x$$
$$2y + 2x = 7y - 3x$$
$$5x = 5y$$

and $\qquad x = y$

so that dividing by $y - x$ is dividing by zero (not allowed in algebra).

C.2.1. 0.6, 0.8

C.2.2. 1, 0

C.2.3. 10

C.2.4. 20

C.3.1. a. 1; b. −1; c. 2; d. −3

C.3.2. a. 5.5×10^4

b. 4.22×10^8

c. 5×10^{-3}

d. 8.2×10^{-8}

C.4.1. 20

C.4.2. 10

C.4.3. 40

C.4.4. −10, 10

C.4.5. 20, 4

C.4.6. 32

C.4.7. 0.003

C.4.8. 1.9

C.4.9. 45, 32,000

C.4.10. −2, 2, 0.63

C.5.1. two (0,1)

C.5.2. bit

C.5.3. two (off, on)

C.5.4. a. 3; b. 7; c. 8; d. 5; e. 4; f. 2; g. 1; h. 6

C.5.5. 25

C.5.6. 1101

C.5.7. a. 5; b. 10; c. 3; d. 1; e. 9; f. 2; g. 8; h. 7; i. 4; j. 6

C.5.8. a. 1 (0); b. 1 (1); c. 3 (101); d. 4 (1010); e. 5 (11001); f. 5 (11110); g. 6 (111111); h. 7 (1000000); i. 7 (1001011); j. 7 (1100100)

C.5.9. a. 3 (111); b. 4 (1111); c. 2 (11); d. 9 (111111111); e. 10 (1111111111); f. 6 (111111); g. 8 (11111111); h. 1 (1); i. 7 (1111111); j. 5 (11111)

C.5.10. a. 1 (0,1); b. 2 (00,01,10,11); c. 3 (000, 001, 010, 011, 100, 101, 110, 111); d. 4; e. 4; f. 5; g. 5; h. 6; i. 7; j. 7

C.6.1. megahertz, 1000

C.6.2. 0.05, 50,000

C.6.3. 1.5, 1500, 150,000, 1,500,000

C.6.4. 0.5, 0.0005, 0.0000005

C.6.5. b

C.6.6. d

C.6.7. c

Appendix D

D.1.1. direction
D.1.2. increased
D.1.3. force
D.1.4. mass
D.1.5. position
D.1.6. velocity
D.1.7. force, mass, acceleration
D.1.8. compression
D.1.9. 2.5
D.1.10. 10
D.1.11. 25
D.1.12. 0.5
D.1.13. 0.2 (pressure is not needed for the calculation)
D.1.14. 25
D.1.15. 3, west

D.2.1. a. 5; b. 2; c. 6; d. 7; e. 3; f. 8; g. 1; h. 4; i. 10; j. 9
D.2.2. work
D.2.3. work
D.2.4. heat
D.2.5. energy
D.2.6. 24, 48
D.2.7. 1250, 31
D.2.8. doubled, quadrupled
D.2.9. doubled, doubled
D.2.10. voltage, current, resistance
D.2.11. power
D.2.12. b, d, e
D.2.13. 50
D.2.14. 50
D.2.15. 12
D.2.16. 2, 2
D.2.17. 2

References

1. Kremkau FW: Education in the physics of diagnostic ultrasound: Is it necessary? Appl Radiol 10:112, 1981
2. Kremkau FW: Technical topics (a column appearing bimonthly in the Reflections section). J Ultrasound Med, vol 2, 1983, through vol 3, 1984
3. Kremkau FW: Physical principles review (a regularly appearing column). Med Ultrasound, vol 4, 1980, through vol 8, 1984
4. Kremkau FW: Physics: What every clinician should know (UM 15), and Principles of real-time cardiac imaging (UM 17). Slide/audio cassette programs. Bethesda, MD, American Institute of Ultrasound in Medicine, 1981
5. Zweibel WJ: Physics. Semin Ultrasound 4:1–62, 1983
6. McDicken WN: Diagnostic Ultrasonics: Principles and Use of Instruments. New York, John Wiley & Sons, 1981
7. Wells PNT, Ziskin MD (eds): Clinics in Diagnostic Ultrasound, vol 5: New Techniques and Instrumentation in Ultrasonography. New York, Churchill Livingstone, 1980
8. Wells PNT: Biomedical Ultrasonics. New York, Academic Press, 1977
9. Edmonds PD, Dunn F: Introduction: Physical description of ultrasonic fields, in Edmonds, PD (ed): Ultrasonics. Methods of Experimental Physics, vol 19. New York, Academic Press, 1981
10. Goss SA, Johnson RL, Dunn F: Comprehensive compilation of empirical ultrasonic properties of mammalian tissues. J Acoust Soc Am 64:423–457, 1978; 68:93–108, 1980

276

11. Carson PL, Fischella PR, Oughton TV: Ultrasonic power and intensities produced by diagnostic ultrasound equipment. Ultrasound Med Biol 3:341–350, 1978

12. Nyborg WL: Ultrasonic intensities generated by real-time devices, in Winsberg F, Cooperberg PL (eds): Clinics in Diagnostic Ultrasound, vol 10: Real-time Ultrasonography. New York, Churchill Livingstone, 1982, pp 15–17

13. Barnett SB, Kossoff G: Ultrasonic exposure in static and real-time echography. Ultrasound Med Biol 8:273–276, 1982

14. Kremkau FW: Ultrasound instrumentation: Physical principles, in Callen PW (ed): Ultrasonography in Obstetrics and Gynecology. Philadelphia, WB Saunders, 1982, pp 313–324

15. Hunter TB, Haber K: A comparison of real-time scanning with conventional static B-mode scanning. J Ultrasound med 2:363–368, 1983

16. Cooperberg P: Real-time ultrasound of the abdomen: Clinical usefulness and limitation. Appl Radiol 9:130, 1980

17. Merritt CRB, Foreman M, Bluth EI, et al: Clinical application of real-time. Appl Radiol 10:83, 1981

18. Laing FC: Commonly encountered artifacts in clinical ultrasound. Semin Ultrasound 4:27–43, 1983

19. Goldstein A: Quality Assurance in Diagnostic Ultrasound. Bethesda, MD, American Institute of Ultrasound in Medicine, 1980

20. Carson PL, Dubuque GL: Ultrasound instrument quality control procedure. Chevy Chase, MD, American Association of Physicists in Medicine, 1980

21. Banjavic RA: Design and maintenance of a quality assurance program for diagnostic ultrasound equipment. Semin Ultrasound 4:10–26, 1983

22. Kremkau FW: How safe is obstetric ultrasound? Contemp OB/GYN 20:182–186, 1982

23. Kremkau FW: Biological effects and possible hazards, in Campbell S (ed): Ultrasound in Obstetrics and Gynaecology. London, WB Saunders, 1983, pp 395–405

24. Kremkau FW: Safety and long-term effects of ultrasound: What to tell your patients, in Platt LD (ed): Perinatal Ultrasound. Clin Obstet Gynecol 27:269–275, 1984

25. Nyborg WL: Physical mechanisms for biological effects of ultrasound. DHEW publications (FDA) 78-8062. Rockville, MD, US Food and Drug Administration, 1977

26. Nyborg WL: Biophysical mechanisms of ultrasound, in Repacholi MH, Benwell DA (eds): Essentials of Medical Ultrasound. Clifton NJ, Humana Press, 1982

27. American Institute of Ultrasound in Medicine: Communication from the AIUM Bioeffects Committee. J Clin Ultrasound 5:2–4, 1977

28. American Institute of Ultrasound in Medicine: Statement on Mammalian in vivo Ultrasonic Biological Effects. Reflections 4:311, 1978

29. American Institute of Ultrasound in Medicine: AIUM Bioeffects Committee. J Ultrasound Med 2:R14, 1983

30. AIUM Evaluation of Biological Effects Research Reports. Bethesda, MD, American Institute of Ultrasound in Medicine, 1984

31. Safety Considerations for Diagnostic Ultrasound. Bethesda, MD, American Institute of Ultrasound in Medicine, 1984

32. AIUM-NEMA Safety Standard for Diagnostic Ultrasound Equipment. Bethesda, MD, American Institute of Ultrasound in Medicine, 1981

33. American Institute of Ultrasound in Medicine: AIUM Safety Statements. J Ultrasound Med 2:R69, 1983

34. American Institute of Ultrasound in Medicine: Statement on Clinical Safety. J Ultrasound Med 3:R10, 1984

35. Kinsler LE, Frey AR: Fundamentals of Acoustics. New York, John Wiley & Sons, 1962, Fig 7.9

36. Zemanek J: Beam behavior within the near field of a vibrating piston. J Acoust Soc Am 49:181–191, 1971

37. Acoustical Terminology. USA Standard ANSI S1.1-1960 (R-1976). New York, American National Standards Institute, 1960

38. Recommended Nomenclature: Physics and Engineering. Bethesda, MD, American Institute of Ultrasound in Medicine, 1979

39. Zweibel WJ: Review of basic terms used in diagnostic ultrasound. Semin Ultrasound 4:60–62, 1983

Index

Absorption, defined, 23
Acceleration, defined, 267
Acoustic output, 163–164
    in diagnostic ultrasound
        instruments, 77–79
Acoustic propagation, defined, 1–2
Acoustic speckle, defined, 4
Acoustic variables
    defined, 5
    propagation speed and, 8
AIUM (American Institute of
        Ultrasound in Medicine),
        155, 158, 167, 174–175
AIUM 100-m test object, 155
Algebra, concepts and exercises in,
        243–249
Alternating voltage, from
        continuous-wave sound, 51
Ambiguity, as artifact, 148–149
American Institute of Ultrasound in
        Medicine (AIUM), 155. See
        also AIUM
Amplification
    attenuation compensation and, 82
    defined, 80
Amplifier
    gain of, 80
    power ratio for, 84

Amplitude absorption coefficient,
        units for, 182
Amplitude, defined, 18–19
Amplitude-mode operation, 98–99
Amplitude reflection, impedance
        difference and, 180
Analog scan converter, 88–89, 92
Angle of incidence, see Incidence
        angle
Angular resolution, 65
Annular array, 113
Annular phased array, 114–115
Artifacts, 139–153
    ambiguity, 148–149
    causes of, 139–140
    defined, 139
    effective reflecting area and, 141
    lateral and axial resolution
        limitations in, 140
    mirror-image, 144–146
    motion, 149
    multiple reflections or
        reverberations in, 140
    propagation speed error as, 146
    reflector positioning and,
        145–147
    refraction as, 144
    side-view reflections as, 145

280

Artifacts, *continued*
    types of, 140, 193
    useful, 139
Attenuation
    defined, 23
    equation for, 23, 25
    image depth and, 25
    intensity and, 24
    in lung tissue, 25
    path length and, 80
    reflections and, 82
    for soft tissues, 23
Attenuation coefficient, 23
    average, 24
    for in vitro tissue samples, 187
    in tissues, 24
Attenuation compensation, by
    varying amplification, 82
Attenuation gain, decibel values of,
    255
Axial resolution
    equation for, 64
    frequency and, 64–65, 69
    half-intensity depth and, 65
    as lateral resolution, 69
    measurement of, 156
    reflector separation and, 66–67
Azimuthal resolution, 65

Backscatter, defined, 43
Backscatter intensity, variations in,
    43
Bandwidth
    defined, 53
    versus frequency, 54
    frequency range and, 188
Beam, for flat disc transducer
    element, 179
Beam area, equation for, 57
Beam cross section, measurement
    of, 162
Beam diameter. *See also* Sound
    beams
    defined, 56
    versus disc diameter, 179
    in focal region, 59
    lateral resolution and, 65
    for single-element disc transducer,
    58

Beam profile, 160–162
Beam profiler, defined, 160
Beam steering, with linear phased
    array, 118
Beam uniformity ratio, 19
Beam width, slice thickness artifacts
    and, 140
Bidirectional instrument, Doppler
    shift and, 128
Binary numbers, 256–260
Bioeffects, 166–172
    mechanism of action in, 170–171
    information sources on, 167–168
Biological Effects Committee,
    AIUM, 167
Bistable display, 105
Bits, in digital memories, 91. *See
    also* Binary numbers
B-mode image, buildup of, 104. *See
    also* B-scan operation
Bone, propagation speed in, 9
Brightness-mode operation, 99
B-scan instruments, misconceptions
    about, 178–179
B-scan operation, 99
B-scan presentation, of reflection,
    103

Cathode-ray tube
    design of, 98
    spot deflection on, 99
Characteristic acoustic impedance,
    defined, 188
Clock or timing circuit, 189–190
Compensation, defined, 80
Compensation operation,
    measurement of, 158
Compressibility, defined, 268
Compression
    defined, 82–84
    function of, 84
Computer memories, 88. *See also*
    Memory
Continuous mode, transducer
    operation on, 49
Continuous-wave, defined, 13
Continuous-wave
    Doppler measurements,
    128–133

instruments, Doppler shift and, 128–133
mode transducer, 49
sound, conversion to alternating voltage, 51
Conversion factors, conversion units and, 262
Coupling media, 34
Curved reflector, 141–143

Dead zone
defined, 156
in imaging performance, 155
Decibel, defined, 82
Decibel gain, intensity ratio and, 255
Demodulation
defined, 82
in digital processing, 95
Density
defined, 267
propagation speed and, 180
Density difference, reflection and, 181
Depth of image, pulse repetition frequency and, 147–149
Depth resolution, 64
Detection, defined, 82
Diagnostic ultrasound. See also Ultrasound
acoustic outputs in, 77–79
bioeffects of, 166–172, 193
misconceptions and errors about, 178–191
pulse–echo, 44
safety of, 172–175
Diagnostic ultrasound parameters, in tissue, 28
Diagnostic ultrasound visualization method, 3. See also Imaging performance
Digital memories
bits in, 91
characteristics of, 90
gray-scale resolution and, 95
10 × 10 pixel, 91
Digital postprocessing, defined, 93
Digital preprocessing, defined, 92
Digital scan converter, 88–90

Disc transducer, beams for, 58–63, 179. See also Transducer(s)
Disc transducer element, 50
Displacement, defined, 267
Display nodes, 98
Displays, 98–107
range marker dots in, 105
television monitors for, 105
videotape recording of, 105
Doppler effect, 123–124
Doppler instruments, 123–136
continuous or pulsed voltages and, 128
real-time and pulsed, 133
Doppler shift, 123
bidirectional instruments and, 128
equation for, 125, 191
negative, 126
production of, 192
propagation speed and, 191
scatter speeds of, 126–127
sound propagation angle and, 125
Doppler-shifted frequencies, return of to transducer, 134
Duty factor
for continuous sound, 20
defined, 15
Dynamic B-mode display, production of, 113
Dynamic focusing, 113
Dynamic imaging, 112
instruments for, 112–122
Dynamic range, defined, 84

Echo-free region, misconceptions about, 179
Echo intensity, 92
Echo pulses, overlapping, 190
Effective reflecting area, artifacts and, 141
Electrical voltages, ultrasound in production of, 48
Electric current, defined, 269–270
Electricity, defined, 269
Electric power, defined, 270
Electric resistance, defined, 270
Electronic noise, elimination of, 85
Energy concepts, 269–270

Energy, defined, 269
Enhancement artifact, 139
Envelope detection, defined, 82
Equations, list of, 239–242

Far zones, sound beams and, 57
Fluid-filled lung, misconception
    about, 183
Focal length, in sound focusing,
    60
Focal region
  of beam, 189
  beam diameter and, 59
Focusing, of sound, 59–61
Force, defined, 266
Fractional bandwidth, defined, 53
Fractional volume change, defined,
    267
Frame, defined, 120
Frame imaging, information storage
    and, 88
Frame rate, pulse repetition
    frequency and, 120
Frequency
  axial resolution and, 64–65
  bandwidth and, 54
  defined, 6–7
  half-intensity depth and, 64–65
  period and, 7
  propagation speed and, 187
  pulse repetition, 120
  within pulses, 187
Frequency range, useful, 64–68
Frequency spectrum plot, 135
Fresnel zone, 56

Gain, defined, 80. See also
    Amplification
Generator gate, of pulsed Doppler
    instrument, 131
Gray-scale display, 105
  beam cross section measurement
    on, 162
Gray-scale dynamic range, defined,
    158
Gray-scale resolution, of digital
    memories, 93–95

Half-intensity depth
  axial resolution and, 65
  frequency and, 64–65
  in tissue, 27
Heart cycle, spectral analysis in,
    134–135
Heat, defined, 269
Hertz, defined, 6
Hydrophones
  as beam profilers, 160
  defined, 163

Image memories, types of, 88
Imaging
  dynamic, 112–122
  static, 88. See also Static imaging
    instruments
Imaging depth
  attenuation and, 25
  equation for, 188
Imaging performance, 154–159
  measurement of, 193
  parameters in, 154–155
  registration accuracy in, 155
Imaging systems
  components of, 74–75, 193
  pulse–echo, 75–78
  visual displays for, 74
Impedance, defined, 10, 34
Impedance difference, amplitude
    reflection and, 180–181
Incidence
  oblique, see Oblique incidence
  perpendicular, see Perpendicular
    incidence
Incidence angle
  intensity reflection coefficient
    and, 183–185
  in oblique incidence, 37
  reflection amplitude and, 182
  reflection angle and, 40, 182
  transmission angles for, 39
Incident intensity, 32
Intensity
  versus amplitude, 18
  defined, 18–19
  equation for, 18, 25, 187
  incident, 32

SATP, 20
SPTA, 20
SPTP, 21
temporal average, 20
versus time, 20
Intensity ratio, 25
decibel gain and, 255
Intensity reflection coefficient
defined, 32
equation for, 33, 35
incidence angle and, 183–185
Intensity transmission coefficient,
defined, 32

Lateral Resolution
beam diameter and, 65
defined, 65
measurement of, 157
reflector separation and, 68–69
Linear array, 113
Linearly translating transducer, 114
Linear phased array, 113–114
beam steering with, 118
operation of, 117
variable focusing with, 118
Linear switched array, 113
operation of, 116
Logarithmic amplifiers, 82–84
Logarithms, in mathematics, 251–
254
Longitudinal resolution, 64
Lung tissue, attenuation in, 25

Mass, defined, 267
Mathematics, review of, 243–265
Maximum imaging depth, lines per
frame and, 148–149
Mechanics, concepts in, 266–269
Media impedances, and absence of
reflection, 181
Megahertz, defined, 6
Memory, 88–95
digital, 90–95
Doppler shift information storage
in, 129–130
types of, 88
Millisecond, defined, 13

Mirror image artifact, 144–146
M-mode display, recording of, 105
Mode presentation, of reflection,
100–101
Motion artifacts, 149
Motion-mode operation, 99
Multipath artifacts, 144
Multiple reflections
as artifacts, 140–141
generation of, 142

Near-zone length
equation for, 56, 59
for unfocused transducers, 59
Newton's second law, 268
NZL, see Near-zone length

Oblique incidence, 32
defined, 37
refraction and, 46, 192
Oblique reflection, 141–143
Ohm's law, 270
Operating frequency, of transducer,
50. See also Frequency
Oscillating mirror, 114
Oscillating transducer, 114

Panel controls, in postprocessing,
93
Particle motion, 5
Performance, imaging, see Imaging
performance
Performance measurements, 154–
165
Perpendicular incidence
defined, 32
reflection and, 46, 192
reflection and transmission at
boundary with, 34
Phased array, 113. See also Linear
phased array
operation of, 117
Physics concepts, 266–271
Piezoelectricity, in ultrasound
transducers, 49

284

Pixel
defined, 88
in digital memories, 91
in memory matrix, 92
Postprocessing assignment schemes, 94–95
Postprocessing, defined, 92–93
Potentiometers, on scan arm necks, 102–104
Power, defined, 269
Power ratio
decibel gain and, 255
defined, 80, 84
Preamplifier, function of, 80
Preprocessing, defined, 92
Pressure reflection, impedance difference and, 180–181
Probe, transducer assembly as, 49–50
Propagation speed
in bone, 9
defined, 9
versus density, 180
density and stiffness factors in, 8
Doppler shift and, 191
frequency and, 187
impedance and, 34
of pulses, see Pulse repetition frequency
in specific tissues, 9–10
of wavelength, 8
Propagation speed error artifacts, 146–147
Pulse, see Pulsed ultrasound, Ultrasound pulse
Pulsed Doppler instrument, 131
receiver gate in, 132
Pulsed ultrasound, 13
frequency range in, 192
pulse repetition frequency and, 192
transducers in, 51
Pulse duration
defined, 14, 187
duty factor and, 15
Pulse–echo diagnostic ultrasound, range equation and, 44–46.
See also Pulsed ultrasound

Pulse–echo imaging
components in, 75
displays in, 193
timing sequence in, 78
Pulse–echo information collection method, 75
Pulse frequency, quality factor and, 53
Pulser
electric voltage pulses for, 77
in pulse–echo imaging system, 75
Pulse repetition frequency
defined, 13–14
equation for, 147
frame rate and, 120
pulse duration and, 192
Pulse repetition period, defined, 13–14
Pulses, propagation speed for, 16.
See also Propagation speed

Quality factor, equation for, 53

Range accuracy
measurement of, 156
testing of, 157
Range equation, 44–46
Range resolution, 64
Rayl, defined, 10
Real-time
displays, 120
imaging, advantages of, 112–113
transducers, 113–119. See also Transducer(s)
Receiver(s), 79–87
functions of, 79, 86, 193
gain and, 80
Receiver gate, of pulsed Doppler instrument, 132–133
Reflecting area, effective, 141
Reflection, 32–42
absence of, 181
B-scan presentation of, 103
density differences and, 181
mode presentation of, 100–101
oblique, 141–143

perpendicular incidence and, 46
presentations of, 100–102
specular, 42
voltage amplitude and, 82
weak, 155
Reflection amplitude, 80
increasing incidence angle and,
182
Reflection angle
incidence angle and, 40
in oblique incidence, 37
Reflection coefficients
calculation of, 40
equal, 80–81
Reflection intensity, 32
Reflector
curved, 141–143
depth, reflection amplitude and,
80
improper positioning of, 145–147
reflection coefficient of, 80–81
roughness, 141–144
separation, in axial resolution,
67–69
Refraction
as artifact, 144
defined, 38
oblique incidence and, 46
Registration accuracy
in imaging performance, 155
test for, 158–159
Registration, defined, 158
Rejection, defined, 85
Relative system sensitivity, 155
Resolution, 64–69
Resonance frequency, 50
Reverberations, generation of, 142
Rod groups(s)
in axial resolution measurement,
156
in compensation operation
measurement, 158
in range accuracy testing, 157

SATA (spatial-average–temporal-
average) intensity, 20
conversion factor for, 21

SATP (spatial-average–temporal-
peak) intensity, conversion
factor for, 21
Scan converters, 105
memory and, 88
Scan line, 98
Scanning
arrays and, 133
real-time transducers in, 113
Scanning arm, articulated,
102–104
Scatterer, defined, 43–45
Scattering, 23, 42–44
cause of, 43
incident sound and, 43
multiple, 85
at rough boundaries, 192
Scientific notation, 251–255
Sensitivity, uniformity, and axial
resolution test, 159
Shadowing artifact, 139
Side lobes, sound beams and, 56
Side-view reflections, as artifacts,
145
Single-element disc transducer
beam diameter and, 58
sound beam for, 56
Snell's law, 38, 182
correct form of, 188
Soft tissues. See also Tissue(s)
attenuation for, 23
spatial pulse length for, 15
Sound
defined, 5–6
parameters of, 5–6
propagation speed of, 6
Sound beams, 56–62. See also
Beam
area units in, 18, 57
diameter of, 56
for disc transducers, 58–63
far zone in, 57
focusing of, 18, 59–61
near zone in, 56
from single-element transducer,
56
Sound direction, axial resolution
and, 64

286

Sound focusing, 18, 59–61
  by curved transducer, 61
Sound source, operating frequency
  of, 18
Sound wave
  defined, 5
  frequency of, 6
  propagation of, 8
Spatial average intensity, equation
  for, 19
Spatial pulse length, defined, 15–16
Speckle, acoustic, 44
Spectral analysis, 134–136
  heart cycle in, 135
Specular reflections, 42
Speed error artifacts, 139
SPTA (spatial-peak–temporal-
  average) intensity, 20
  conversion factor for, 21
SPTP (spatial-peak–temporal-peak)
  intensity, 20
  conversion factor for, 21
Static imaging, echo information
  storage in, 88
Static imaging instruments, 74–111
Static scanning, versus dynamic,
  112
Stationary transducer, 114
Stiffness, defined, 267
SUAR test, 159
Suppression, defined, 85
Symbols, list of, 237–238

Television monitors, for displays,
  105
Temperature, defined, 269
Temporal average intensity,
  equation for, 20
Tissue(s)
  acoustic propagation properties
    of, 2
  attenuation coefficients in, 24
  average attenuation coefficients
    in, 24
  average half-intensity depths in,
    27
  diagnostic ultrasound parameters
    in, 28

multiple scattering in, 85
propagation speed in, 9–10
soft, see Soft tissues
ultrasound interaction with, 166
ultrasound periods and
  wavelengths in, 8
Tissue-equivalent phantoms, 158
Tissue parenchyma, 42
  scattering in imaging of, 43
Transducer(s), 48–56. See also
  Ultrasound transducers
  in diagnostic ultrasound
    visualization, 3
  discs as, 49–50
  examples of, 49
  function of, 71
  in pulse–echo imaging system, 75
  pulsed sound and, 13
  on scanning arm, 102
  in ultrasound parameter
    determination, 76
Transducer arrays, defined, 113
Transducer assembly, 49–50
  in pulsed mode, 52
Transducer element, 49
  voltage pulse applied to, 53
Transducer face, matching layer on,
  52
Transducer types, 114
Transmission angle, in oblique
  incidence, 37
Transverse resolution, 65
Trigonometry, concepts and
  exercises in, 299
Two-frequency disc transducers,
  beam diameters for, 60

Ultrasound. See also Sound
  bioeffects of, 166–172
  defined, 1
  diagnostic, see Diagnostic
    ultrasound
  frequency of, 5
  mammalian effects of, 167–171
  risk–benefit information on, 167,
    173
  safety of, 166, 172–175
  tissues and, see Tissue(s)

Ultrasound imaging, scattering in, 43. *See also* Imaging
Ultrasound parameters, determination of, 76
Ultrasound pulse. *See also* Pulsed ultrasound
  diameter of, 57
  generation of, 56
Ultrasound transducers. *See also* Transducer(s)
  defined, 48–49
  as discs, 49–50
  function of, 71
  near-zone length for, 59
  piezoelectricity in, 49
  in pulsed mode, 51
  single-element, 49
Units
  conversion factors for, 262
  for physics and acoustic quantities, 260–265
Useful frequency range, 64–68

Variable focusing, with linear phased array, 118
Velocity
  defined, 182, 267
  units for, 182, 260
Voltage generator
  of continuous-wave Doppler instrument, 128
  of pulsed Doppler instrument, 131–133
Voltage pulses
  from pulser, 77
  from source transducers, 51
  for transducer element, 53

Wave. *See also* Sound wave
  longitudinal, 5
  power in, 18
Wavelength(s)
  defined, 6–7
  equation for, 8
  list of, 8
Work, defined, 269